INSPIRED TO FEEL GOOD

Praise for the Book

"Alice provides a whole new way to think and feel about eating, being active and improving your personal health. This book gives you permission to first take care of yourself and make the right lifestyle choices that are inspiring, motivating and enjoyable to maintain for long term health and wellness. You'll be enriched, and I highly recommend it."

—Nick Yphantides, MD, physician and author of *My Big Fat Greek Diet*

"*Inspired to Feel Good* offers a practical and enjoyable approach to healthy eating and regular exercise. The book is filled with success stories and specific strategies that will inspire you to discover your own personal path to wellness."

—Michelle May, MD, physician and author of *Am I Hungry?*

"Alice has brilliantly identified three simple steps to change how you approach your food and fitness that gives you the confidence and control to enjoy your life and feel good about yourself."

—Diana Lipson-Burge, RD, intuitive eating pioneer
and co-author of *Un-Dieting*

"Alice Greene shares her wise and welcome formula for helping you change the way you eat and exercise by helping you change the way you *think* and *feel. Inspired to Feel Good* is a gift."

—Keith Ablow, MD, renowned psychiatrist and author of
Living the Truth and *Inside the Mind of Scott Peterson*

"It takes energy, passion & persistence to succeed in all areas of your life. Alice's book *Inspired to Feel Good* shows you how to find that inner motivation and drive so you will take care of your greatest asset.... YOU! Keep in mind what you put into your head is often more important than what goes in your mouth and Alice shows you how to create affirming beliefs and strategies to help you succeed in your quest for lifelong health. This book makes it possible for everyone to succeed at living a healthier lifestyle."

—John M. Rowley, fitness expert and author of
Climb YOUR Ladder of Success Without Running Out of Gas!

"Alice offers wisdom about how to eat and exercise in this powerful and common sense book that will help you succeed at reaching your health, fitness and weight loss goals. I have worked with Alice personally and highly recommend her unique approach."

—Marcia Wieder, CEO and founder of Dream University®
and author of *Dreams are Whispers from the Soul.*

"*Inspired to Feel Good* succeeds where too many diet and exercise books fail — in supporting lasting, real-life change even in the face of real-life challenges. Alice Greene empowers her readers to embrace sustainable, rewarding shifts in behavior that lead not only to better health, but to great happiness and life satisfaction. This book is enormously wise, well-rounded and a helpful guidance for those looking to make a lasting commitment to health and fitness."

—Pilar Gerasimo, Editor in Chief, Experience Life magazine

INSPIRED TO FEEL GOOD

**Making healthy and fit choices
so rewarding and liberating
you never want to stop**

ALICE GREENE

New York

Inspired to Feel Good

Making Healthy and Fit Choices So Rewarding and Liberating You Never Want to Stop

ISBN 978-1-60037-565-1

Library of Congress Control Number: 2008943791

MORGAN · JAMES
THE ENTREPRENEURIAL PUBLISHER

Morgan James Publishing, LLC
1225 Franklin Ave., STE 325
Garden City, NY 11530-1693
Toll Free 800-485-4943
www.MorganJamesPublishing.com

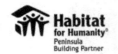

In an effort to support local communities, raise awareness and funds, Morgan James Publishing donates one percent of all book sales for the life of each book to Habitat for Humanity. Get involved today, visit **www.HelpHabitatForHumanity.org.**

To my mother Anna
who has traveled the long journey
beside me with an open mind and loving heart

and

To my clients
who took the leap of faith that changed their lifestyles
and from whom I learned so much

In Gratitude

My heartfelt appreciation and gratitude goes to my dear and loyal friend, Gail Jones, who cheered me on, jumped in to serve as editor and continues to share the road-less traveled while pursuing our purposeful and starlit journeys. She has been my rock and my roll.

I also have enormous gratitude for the trust so many clients put in me, as they opened their mindset to a new way of relating to food, exercise, their bodies and themselves. This book would not have been possible without their willingness to try something new, and from them I witnessed how powerful the gift of self-awareness, self-discovery and self-choice can be in attaining personal freedom and self-love.

Specifically, I want to thank the sixty clients who gave me permission and their blessing to share parts of their story in this book. To ensure their privacy, I have changed their names. I also want to thank the fifteen guests from my radio show who also allowed me to reference part of their healthy lifestyle success stories throughout this book.

There are too many coaching colleagues who have shaped my thinking and work to mention, yet there are a few who have been instrumental in my growth and practice I do wish to acknowledge. To all the times we persevered, did what it took and kept the faith, I am forever grateful to Ann Seelye, Amy Lundberg, Lisa Atkinson, Gillian Hood-Gabrielson and Heather Moreno. Our passion for this work is the fuel that drives us.

I also want to thank John Rowley and David Hancock who saw the potential in me and championed my efforts to get this book out into the world.

Table of Contents

Introduction

Introduction

Barbara knew how good it felt to be active and to eat healthy foods, but she had reached a point where she didn't care anymore. It had been more than a year since she had gone to Curves regularly, and she was beginning to think it didn't really matter if she ever went back. Two years before, she had been serious about taking better care of herself after learning she had high cholesterol and was at risk for diabetes and heart disease. Yet she struggled to stick with her improved eating habits and exercise routine, and she eventually succumbed to the inertia of doing nothing. She had tried other programs, worked with trainers and tried Weight Watchers in the past, but none of these regimens worked for her. She wanted help, but she wasn't sure where or whom to get it from.

When we first talked, Barbara told me she didn't feel very well. Her body ached, her knee bothered her and she just didn't feel good. She wanted to feel better, get past her ambivalence about taking care of herself and find a way to be motivated to make fitness a way of life. She had succeeded in being regularly active after undergoing a hip replacement many years before and knew she could do it again. Yet she also told me, "I don't have it in me to do this right now, and I have a sense of failing and hopelessness."

Despite feeling despondent, she decided to work with me for a while and see if she could recapture her zest for healthy living and reduce her risk of disease. Barbara started off easy, choosing aerobic exercise three times a week by either walking or doing a Richard Simmons video. She discovered that it felt good to be in motion again. She realized that although she had put off exercise, once she got moving, her mood lifted, and it felt wonderful to get her heart rate up. Within six weeks she was also going to Curves twice a week, and her knee, which had bothered her for years, wasn't so painful anymore. By the eighth week of her new routine, she was really seeing some big shifts in how she felt. In our eighth session, she said, "It was like old times this week. I got a great feeling from exercising. It really feels good, and my body wants to do it. I feel secure trusting in my body and myself, and I feel balanced."

Barbara also began changing the way she looked at food. She learned to listen to her hunger signals and to eat whenever she got hungry and to stop eating when she was satisfied but not full. She also discovered that it wasn't so hard to eat more vegetables or to prepare nutritionally balanced meals and snacks so she had food available whenever she got hungry. By the sixth week, she was finding she really liked eating healthy meals and was feeling better physically. And she told me, "Every time I don't eat a healthy meal, I naturally gravitate back to healthy options without bingeing. I'm not out of control. With balanced meals, I'm not obsessed or getting too hungry. I'm also gaining trust in having some of my 'forbidden foods' in moderation."

She was learning it wasn't about judging herself for eating the right or wrong foods, but about getting clear on the underlying issues that were driving her eating behaviors that mattered. When you can be conscious of your behavior, such as choosing unhealthy food or overeating, without judging it, you can stop for a moment to check in with yourself and see what is driving your choices. At that point you can decide if it is the food you really need or something else. Barbara had an epiphany in the eighth week. She told me, "This is so much more than about food [and she's right]. Without controlling everything, I have more control, and it is less about judging things as good or bad but accepting there is no perfect way." Within the next couple of weeks, she was happier, more confident, and trusting herself to make choices that served her better. She also noticed that the less she judged her behavior with food, the less she judged herself and others elsewhere in her life. By the twelfth week of following this program, she was feeling like she was really living life and not depriving herself or feeling hung up about food. She claimed, "I know what I'm hungry for and how I can balance it, which makes eating flow so easily." She was now in control and feeling free to really enjoy food without the fear of being preoccupied by it or of judging herself.

When I asked her for a testimonial, this is what she wrote: "This is the missing piece. I already knew about nutrition, diet and exercise, but this self-honoring approach allows me to use all that as part of a lifestyle with greater trust in myself. What is so different is that the focus is on making choices that best serve me instead of trying to measure up to a structure and feeling judged for how well I did. This program helps you trust and feel good about yourself, and I am so thankful for the changes in my thinking. It isn't about fixing me. It is about self-acceptance and having choice. I now feel better, happier and more confident. I also know that I do have control and can keep doing this lifestyle for myself."

Breaking Free of Ambivalence

Barbara's experience of feeling despondent isn't unusual. The feeling of hopelessness also creates a feeling of ambivalence about making healthier choices and feeling better. Right now, probably half of all Americans and nearly as many others around the world are feeling the same way or are looking for a better answer to getting and staying fit and healthy.

Ambivalence makes it difficult to start or keep up a healthy and fit lifestyle. This feeling of both wanting and resisting healthy changes occurs frequently when you are depressed or stressed or have experienced repeated failures in dieting or sticking with a fitness or nutrition program. In time, ambivalence leads to indifference, becoming apathetic and choosing to avoid awareness of your body because of disappointment, shame or feeling overwhelmed. Most people will drift in and out of their indifferent state, often staying apathetic for months or years at a time.

It takes hope, resolve and enough obvious benefit to break free of ambivalence. That usually happens when a defining moment occurs and you are driven to make a lifestyle change. At that point there is a shift out of inertia into taking some type of action, but determining how to shift is where people are getting stuck. Many have come to realize that dieting doesn't work, and they question if going back to the gym or doing the fitness programs available to them will have a better outcome or feel more motivating than the last time they tried them.

A history of yo-yo exercising and dieting can lead people to feel leery of repeating programs or recommendations that haven't worked for them in the past. I hear this repeatedly from my clients who have done dozens of diets and tried many different fitness programs. They don't have the confidence they will succeed or that the programs will really work for them, yet they know they have to do something.

And these people won't succeed without changing their thinking about and approach to being fit and healthy. What gets in the way of success is the mental and emotional mindset that creates your attitude and feelings about making a healthy change and sticking with it as a way of life.

Your current mindset stems from past dieting and fitness experiences and perceptions of yourself and your abilities. It also stems from trying to measure up to someone else's expectations that may be unattainable, aiming for specific weight loss results in a short period of time, or striving to reach unrealistic goals, such as exercising six days a week for a minimum of 45 minutes when you normally do three days at 30 minutes or less, and then seeing yourself as bad or having failed if you don't fully comply or succeed. If you feel achieving anything less than 100 percent or straight As is not good enough or worth doing, it creates the belief that anything less than perfection isn't good enough or you aren't good enough to succeed. This creates all or nothing and good or bad thinking. Believing there is no middle ground, you will eventually give up and berate yourself for not succeeding once again, even if you had successes along the way.

What I am here to show you is how you can reach your goals in the short and long-term in a way that frees you of believing you are bad, wrong or guilty. This is possible with an approach that feels good from the start and is appealing, positive and energizing to keep you motivated along the way to creating a more active and healthier life. Improving your lifestyle doesn't take force and willpower when you are doing and eating healthy things you enjoy in a way that is realistic, reinforcing and empowering.

Feeling So Good You Never Want to Stop

When people call me for coaching, they typically ask for help with losing weight, staying motivated, having some accountability for their goals and sticking with their new behaviors, pretty much in that order. Yet what they really want, I find when we talk further, is to feel better. It is so easy to focus on weight loss and being compliant with a diet or fitness program because of our culture, but what really matters is how you feel physically in your body and how you feel emotionally about yourself.

This book isn't about how to lose weight or how to have enough willpower to eat right and exercise six days a week. This book is about how to create a healthy lifestyle you can't wait to experience because it frees you to explore what feels really good physically, mentally, emotionally and even spiritually. This approach is the opposite of encouraging you to once again comply with rigid guidelines and avoids the inevitable inability to stick with them that leads to self-criticism, emotional eating, weight gain and loss of self-esteem. Instead, the book gives you the guidance and freedom to discover what works and feels good to you at a pace you can live with.

Have you ever tried something new and felt it was easier than you thought, and then become excited because you could do it? When that happened, could you then see why you would want to do more of it? Some people discover this when they first start cooking, gardening, sailing or painting. I don't think too many people say that when they first start working out or dieting. But I will show you a new way to discover the pleasure of being more fit and eating healthier that really is easier than you would expect and that you won't want to stop. As you experience how good the process feels, you will gravitate to making even more healthy changes on your own. You won't need willpower because you will be helping yourself make choices that work for you and your life on your own terms.

What I will share with you will change your relationship with food, fitness, your body and yourself in a way that feels good and natural to you because it won't be forced on you. It will instead validate you and be driven by your own desire and motivation to change in alignment with your values, dreams and needs — and it won't be as difficult as you may expect.

You may wonder, as many of my clients have, why you weren't told what I'm going to share with you before. You may feel angry that you've had to suffer for so long before finding out that reaching your goals didn't have to be so hard and painful. You have a right to those feelings. Sadly, the reason none of us knew this before is because of our culture. Our society promotes the belief that more is better, you have to feel pain to get results and you have to work hard to succeed. Yet you will find less *is* more — that less pain, suffering and work will bring you far greater results.

How I Became a Healthy Lifestyle Success Story and Coach

I didn't know what I know now back in 2000. I was on the verge of a midlife crisis and dealing with high stress, chronic back pain, chronic fatigue and rapid weight gain. I went up four dress sizes the year I was forty-two and another size a couple of months later. My size affected how I felt about myself. I felt embarrassed and was losing my self-esteem. There were times when I felt enormous despair and just wanted to crawl into bed and never come out, which was a feeling I knew well from being overweight and struggling with low self-esteem in my past.

When people meet me, they can't believe I've ever been fat or struggled with health issues. Yet I grew up overeating to compensate for a traumatic childhood and a belief something was wrong with me. Back when I was a child I was called plump, but I felt huge because I was one of the few fat girls in my class and I was so tall. It was humiliating to be fat, and I turned to extreme dieting as a teenager to become thin enough to feel I fit in. This was the beginning of my long history of dieting, which worked to keep me slim and allowed me to avoid serious exercise. I would exercise with great fanfare for a month or so every few years, yet for all practical purposes I was sedentary throughout my twenties and thirties with the exception of a year when I worked with a personal trainer. Unfortunately that was not a positive experience.

Soon after turning forty-three, I had one those defining moments that finally got my attention and put me into action. After being in bed for a couple of months from a repeating episode of chronic fatigue and discovering I didn't fit into the clothes I'd just bought beforehand, I realized enough was enough. I thought if I didn't do something about my health, fitness and weight, it might become too late. I made a pact with myself that day to use the dusty StairMaster aerobic machine in the basement as soon as I was well enough, and I pledged not to quit using it regularly until I could get back into my wardrobe.

I started exercising on January 1, 2001. It was two years before I reached my goal and another year before I discovered I had a passion for fitness and a whole new perspective on living a healthy lifestyle. I also realized I had created a very different method of getting back into shape and reclaiming my health than was typically taught. I had learned how to create and maintain a healthy lifestyle I could happily live with and do my own way, which was exciting. It was also something I thought others would want to know about and could benefit from.

I certainly would have welcomed some healthy lifestyle assistance during those first two years. While I believed I knew what to do for the most part, I wanted some accountability, specific help with my challenges, an expert I could bounce ideas off of, and someone to share my successes with. I didn't want another trainer, and I didn't want to join the gym. There were many things I guessed at that worked and others that didn't, which led to slower results and a couple of injuries.

I believed that other people were going through similar experiences and seeking a more holistic approach to fitness, and my initial research validated my thinking. My vision was to combine wellness and life coaching with a foundation in fitness, nutrition and stress reduction. I found the certification and training programs that allowed me to do just that and created a unique blend of expertise in personal training, nutrition, emotional eating, intuitive eating, lifestyle fitness coaching, wellness coaching and dream fulfillment coaching. Together, these certifications and programs gave me a unique and powerful foundation on which to develop a healthy lifestyle coaching practice. By 2004, I was one of the first to practice fitness coaching by phone, and I was amazed by the power coaching had to change my clients' attitudes from "I can't lose weight, stick with it or succeed" to "I can and I want to be active and eat healthier because it feels so much better. I don't have to be perfect."

What I learned during the first four years of my private coaching practice was the correlation between a client's mindset and his or her success. I increasingly turned to my training in emotional eating to help clients resolve old beliefs and feelings that were getting in the way of their progress. The more I did this, the more success clients had. And this in turn led to an even more powerful and unique approach to healthy lifestyle coaching, which I continue to use today.

I now believe the struggle that keeps people from being healthy and fit is often what they believe about themselves and the emotions they keep repressed. It is this emotional and mental baggage that prevents people from reaching their dreams of feeling and looking their best. By addressing what is going on inside your head, you can change what is happening on the outside.

"When you change the way you look at things, the things you look at change."
—Wayne Dyer

I don't claim to be the absolute authority on fitness, nutrition and stress management. Instead I will give you the tools and guidance to help you make decisions about what is best for you and feels good to you so you can be your own authority and know when you need to turn to local experts for additional help.

What makes me so different is my perspective. I have a unique vantage point because I didn't choose the conventional approach to becoming a personal trainer, dietician or healthcare practitioner. Instead I got the certifications I needed and blended several approaches to become an expert in healthy living, and then I chose to work with clients using a coaching model. This approach worked better than I could have imagined, and within the next ten years, I believe the healthy lifestyle coaching approach will be commonplace in the fitness and healthcare industries.

What You Will Learn in This Book

This book will help you understand why it may have been difficult in the past for you to adopt healthier habits, stick with your programs or stay motivated to reach your goals. You will get a new perspective that will make sense, and you will begin to see what can work for you in a way you didn't think was possible.

The book is divided into three sections.

- Part One: Changing Your Mind about Fitness
- Part Two: A New Way of Thinking about Eating, Exercise and Self-Care
- Part Three: Creating a Healthier Lifestyle That Feels Good

Part One: Changing Your Mind about Fitness

In the first section of the book, you will learn that what you've been told in the past about eating right, getting fit and being healthy may be making it harder for you to succeed at reaching your health and fitness goals. You will discover there are good reasons why you may have struggled with dieting, weight loss, working out, having enough willpower or putting yourself first. And then you will be given an empowering perspective for addressing food and fitness that focuses on the mindset that will allow you to succeed. By changing your mindset, you will gain the freedom to finally discover the pleasure of a healthy and fit lifestyle and the confidence that comes with feeling good inside and out.

Part Two: A New Way of Thinking about Eating, Exercise and Self-Care

This section will introduce you to an easy yet powerful three-step process that will change your entire attitude toward and approach to healthy eating, fitness and taking care of yourself. The steps will give you ah-ha insights about your behaviors toward food, exercise and yourself, an awareness of why you make the choices you do, and how to choose healthier options you can easily live with and feel motivated to stick with for the long-term. Even better, these steps only take a minute to do, and once you start using them you'll find they can be applied to many other aspects of your life.

Part Three: Creating a Healthier Lifestyle That Feels Good
In the last section I will walk you through the process of applying the three steps to being active and eating healthier. You will be given everything you need to get started, feel informed, make smart decisions, stay motivated and be supported as you become more healthy and fit. Along the way I will guide and coach you, which will build your fitness and nutrition knowledge and self-confidence that you can succeed. As you read this section, you will come to integrate this process into your new mindset and you will find it easier to make healthier choices as an extension of yourself.

Many people have already experienced this process by working directly with me, and I am grateful to my clients who so graciously allowed their stories to be part of this book so you too can learn from their experiences. They took a leap of faith when they reached out to me and were willing to try something different to overcome their challenges with food, exercise and putting themselves first. And it changed their lives.

Reclaiming the Power to Feel Your Personal Best

You have an opportunity to release the mental and emotional baggage you carry about specific foods, healthy eating, exercise, being in balance or whatever is keeping you from living the full life you deserve and want. I don't promise you'll completely change your mindset in just one week or even the first month, but with the tools and techniques in this book you can become free of what keeps you from reaching your fitness, weight and health goals the more you use them.

In the place of resistance, ambivalence or striving to do better, you can reclaim the power to choose what feels better to you. What I do promise is that if you pay attention to what motivates you and allow your body to guide you, with the techniques I give you the process will feel easier and more enjoyable. I also promise that the better you feel as you make healthier choices, the more healthy decisions you will make, and the more you will incorporate them into your lifestyle. It doesn't have to be hard to be healthy and fit. Instead, I believe it should be easy and based on what feels good to you and your body.

Are you ready to feel your personal best?

Let's get started by turning the page.
Alice Greene

Part One

Changing Your Mind about Fitness

Changing Your Mind about Fitness

How often do you promise yourself that this time you will really follow through on your diet or exercise program, only to find yourself struggling to meet the goals you set? How does that feel, and what do you tell yourself when this happens? Most likely you feel badly about yourself and question if you are capable of following through. You may beat yourself up for good measure. That not only doesn't help, it reinforces negative beliefs about yourself and drives you to repeat the same behaviors.

Sarah, who called me for help, felt helpless in her struggle to get fit. She said, "I don't know what is wrong with me. I just can't get myself motivated and I've let myself go. And now I hate how I feel and I don't even want to try anymore." She told me how bad she was with food and how she failed at sticking with exercising. She didn't even know if she could ever be good enough to lose all the weight that was making her sick. I told her the issue wasn't about being good enough. It was about finding a way to address fitness differently so that it worked for her and so she wouldn't judge herself as being good or bad.

Millions of people are struggling to find a way to force themselves to get more exercise, eat healthier or make their health a priority, and they aren't finding an easy method that consistently works. Do you ever wonder why so many people are in this struggle and why this wasn't such a problem just thirty years ago? Even fifteen years ago, according to the Centers for Disease Control, less than twenty percent of Americans were more than thirty pounds overweight. Now one-third of the population is obese and two-thirds are overweight.

The biggest difference is our mindset, which determines what we think, believe and feel about being active and healthier. We all have different emotions and beliefs when it comes to fitness, yet many would agree with my client Betsy. She said with frustration and concern, "The thought of going back to the gym makes me want to eat a pint of Ben & Jerry's." Well then, going to the gym is not the right answer for her, although it could be in the future. What worked better for her was an aquatics program with lots of great classes and an atmosphere that felt more comfortable, motivating and energizing. There are lots of other ways to be active when you rethink the definition of exercise.

In this section you will learn that much of what you've been taught about nutrition, fitness and healthy habits is not helping you to successfully make healthy lifestyle changes. In fact, the guidance you've received may be your problem. More experts, including dieticians, now recognize that diets are failing people instead of the belief that people are failing at dieting. They see that the problems with dieting are the extreme restrictions and emphasis on strict compliance.

The same problems exist with most fitness, nutritional and healthcare weight-loss programs. When someone feels forced to make highly restrictive and rigid lifestyle changes, even if they've agreed to them, they will likely resist, rebel and eventually give up. This overbearing emphasis on compliance is getting in the way of successfully creating long-term healthy habits for a great many people. There is a better way of looking at food, exercise and taking care of your health and fitness that is inspiring, engaging and addresses the very things that hold you back. This better way is found in the mindset of people who are naturally active, thin and healthy. These people don't struggle to stay in shape. It comes easily to them, and it can come just as easily to you.

Change Your Mindset and Discover an Easier Way

Given a freer way of looking at healthy habits, you can change how you relate to food, exercise, your body and yourself. In the process you will set yourself free of judgment, gain control of your choices and create a healthier lifestyle you can actually enjoy. You will also discover how it feels to have a body and life you love.

No doubt that sounds too good to be true. With your current mindset that probably doesn't seem possible, but I will show you that it is possible by revealing a whole new way of looking at healthier choices.

And that is what you want, isn't it? You are probably sick of the way you feel, how you treat yourself or the energy it takes to overcome the inertia to change. Most everyone wants to feel energized, invigorated, happy, sexy, healthy and able to live fully. In various informal surveys, people often claim they would do anything — even give their lives — to be slim, fit and more appealing, and the sad fact is most people *are* giving their lives by avoiding what it takes to be healthy and in shape. Are you one of these people?

The good news is there is an easy way to get unstuck. There actually *is* a quick fix, but it isn't one you take or do. It is what you believe, and that fix is painless, surprisingly enjoyable and lasts a lifetime.

Are you ready for a fresh approach? Are you ready to finally succeed? If so, follow me. If not, come back when you are ready. As you will soon discover, success doesn't come when you feel pushed or forced into something you aren't comfortable with, so honor yourself and take the next step when it is right for you.

What Is Getting in Your Way of Succeeding?

We live in a culture that has promoted the very things that has caused us to gain weight, struggle to get fit and feel out of control around food. When that happens, many people also experience low self-esteem and a feeling that something is wrong with them.

Nothing is wrong with you or me. We have drunk the quick-fix Kool-Aid that we now know is poisoned. You aren't alone. Most of us tried it because that was all we were given to drink. What we have been told has steered you down the wrong path and given you the wrong idea of what is supposed to work. We were all once told to follow a low-fat diet, then a low-carb diet as well as hundreds of other diets promoted in the media. Even today, everywhere you turn there are diets, pills, programs, trainers, books, studies and experts offering the slimming answer, and they all differ in what they recommend. Furthermore, despite all these options, two-thirds of the population is still struggling to lose weight. You have to wonder, if the programs and diets are all so good, why is it so few people are succeeding? There are many good reasons for this.

Dieting

One of the main culprits is dieting. Even though most dieters believe diets work *when they are on them*, diets seldom lead to long-term success. According to various informal studies, less than five percent of dieters succeed in keeping off the weight they've lost during a diet for at least two years. The other ninety-five percent, who don't succeed, take a breather between diets, determined that the next time they will stick with it and finally have success.

For those that feel they failed to stick with a diet, know that you didn't fail — the diet failed you. Diets are highly restrictive, and it is inevitable that you will eat something that isn't allowed, which leads you to feel you've blown it or can't stick with it. When you fail at something, it affects how you see yourself and lowers your self-esteem. The more often you diet, the more deeply that belief gets ingrained.

One of my clients shared what failure feels like when she said, "I feel like I've hit bottom. I've done a twelve-step program for food and sugar, but I feel powerless and out of control. I know what I'm doing isn't healthy, but I can't stop. I don't trust myself. I feel like a failure, and I think something is wrong with me."

In addition, the more you diet, the more likely you are to gain even more weight once you stop dieting. This is because dieting lowers your metabolism, increases fat hoarding and creates an insatiable desire for the foods listed as forbidden. So it is natural and to be expected that you will overeat, or even binge, as soon as the diet ends. In the book *Intuitive Eating*, Evelyn Tribole and Elyse Resch describe the insatiable desire to make up for what was denied you as "deprivation backlash," and that is a good name for it.

This backlash of overeating then supplies plenty of extra calories to satisfy the body's need to store fat in case there is another food shortage. The more often there is a shortage, the more fat the body wants to store away to ensure survival. Add to this a slower metabolism after a diet (where the body burns fewer calories than before), and you've got a double-whammy when you start eating normally again. The amount of calories burned off is now much lower, so even normal amounts of food — not including deprivation backlash bingeing — will exceed your metabolic rate.

What if I told you that dieting is a leading cause of obesity? I am not alone in believing this is true. A handful of dieticians, physicians and researchers are beginning to say the same thing as they witness continuing weight gain in those who diet repeatedly.

What intrigues me is that when I ask people if they feel diets work; they all say they've had great success with them. I then find out they have dieted repeatedly. If a diet succeeded, then why did these people have to go back on a diet? Success is maintaining the weight loss indefinitely. But the diet mindset convinces you that you succeeded if you lost any weight at all. How does that help if it doesn't last or turns you into an overeater afterward? That is like saying a cell phone works if it gets a signal, even if it loses the signal repeatedly during your calls or only has a signal in certain areas.

Diets don't work, and until you believe that, you will keep trying them and keep drinking the Kool-Aid. They are addictive because they look like a quick fix, and people around you appear to be succeeding with them. But pay attention to how long these other people keep the weight off and ask them how they feel about having to go back on a diet when they no longer feel so good about their success.

Focusing on the Weight

Another culprit getting in the way of feeling and looking your best is the focus on weight and losing a certain number of pounds. Those that finally lose weight and maintain their new shape discover that what matters to them is not really the weight but their health and fitness. Let me say this again. Getting the body you want isn't about the weight, and focusing on the weight is actually the problem. Elizabeth said it well after discovering how good it felt to get fit: "It is now more about how I feel versus what the scale says. I'm more focused on the goal of accomplishing something other than my weight. And I love how good I feel about myself."

Here is the secret that has eluded you and just about everyone else in your shoes: if your main focus is weight loss and reaching a certain number of pounds, then you will be held captive by the scale, believe your weight is your worth and lose focus on what really matters.

When you are obsessed with reaching a number, you are likely to punish or reward yourself based on what the scale says. You are also likely to become obsessed with food, restricting it when you fail to reach the goal and eating more of it when you succeed. But you have less control over what the scale is going to say than you think. You can be up or down a few pounds on any given day because of what or how much you ate or drank, the extent you were recently active, when you last used the bathroom, how hydrated you are or where you are in your menstrual cycle.

When you step on the scale, it could go either way, up or down, and you have no idea which way it is going to go. You hold your breath and dare to look. The number you see will impact how you feel about yourself and your day — or even your whole week — and even worse, it will impact your behavior. If you see a number you are pleased with, you may think, "Hooray! I don't have to diet or try anymore," and you may give in to temptations or unhealthy habits. You may even think you've been so good you deserve a day off and either overeat as a reward or skip your aerobic plans. On the other hand, if the number goes up and you fail to reach your goal, you may be more restrictive in dieting or work out harder to make up for failing. You may feel so badly that you are driven to eat emotionally. These behaviors are self-defeating. Aren't you exhausted by this? Aren't you sick of being jerked around by a number that only you see?

What you don't realize is the scale lies. It is not an accurate reflection of the type of weight that matters. The only weight that matters is the weight of fat. The rest (water, muscle, bone and other tissues), which is about 70 percent of your weight, isn't the problem and isn't what is keeping you overweight. Unfortunately, the scale can't tell the difference between fat and these other things, and even the body mass index (BMI) doesn't give an accurate view of your body's makeup. Furthermore, it is nearly impossible to put on a pound of fat, or even half a pound, in a day. To add a pound of fat would require that you eat an excess of 3,500 calories, above and beyond the 1,500 – 2,000 calories you are already eating and burning in a day.

If I had my way, we would all throw out our scales. I don't own one, and I haven't weighed myself for a couple of years.

When you focus on healthier habits as a way of life to feel energized, alive, fit, healthy and good about yourself, the weight will take care of itself. The more you love yourself at any weight, the less you will care what your weight is, and the easier it will come off. You may even discover your natural body weight makes you happy, even if it is heavier than you thought you could accept. Accepting yourself at "size healthier, size confident and size ideal," as Queen Latifah and Valerie Bertinelli say in recent Jenny Craig advertisements is what is most important. It is wonderful to see this ideal promoted.

Nearly every woman I've talked with who has successfully achieved a healthy lifestyle tells me that she no longer cares about her actual weight. Unlike for men, who tend to be less bothered by excess weight, this tends to be a significant shift in thinking for women. It is those striving to reach a number or to be perfect, including actresses and models who have become society's ultrathin role models, who are unhappy and obsessed. It is always shocking to hear that a celebrity or a model, who looks about as perfect as anyone could ever be, say she hates her thighs or thinks she's too fat.

It is a paradox: the more you want something outside of yourself, the harder it is to attain. By adopting a healthier lifestyle and removing the focus on weight, the more successful you will be at getting what you really want and being the most beautiful you. A great role model for this mindset is Tyra Banks, who is not only a supermodel but also the host of *America's Next Top Model* and her own talk show. She is out to prove that you don't have to be a size 2 or weigh 115 pounds to be considered sexy, beautiful or a cover girl. She is proud not to be super skinny. At 160 pounds, she is showing women that it is more than okay to fill out our curves and love ourselves for our natural beauty and weight. This was a daring stance to take, and it took courage to stand up to the media backlash she got, but she made her point with grace and is a role model for us all.

Working Out

A culprit you may not expect is the workout and how you feel about it. The idea of a workout represents working hard to burn calories, and it encourages the no-pain-no-gain attitude that leads to injuries, burnout and quitting. When most of us think of doing a workout, we think of gyms, fitness programs or home exercise equipment, and we think of pushing our bodies to the max. We also often think *get in, get out* and focus on how many calories we can burn in a specific number of minutes. This isn't about doing something we look forward to but calculating how soon we can get it behind us so we can be good, burn off our excess calories and say we exercised. This isn't to say all workouts are bad. What can be bad is how we approach them and feel about them.

Let's take this a step further. What is the first thing that comes to mind when you hear the word *exercise*? If you are like most people, you think *working out*. Why is that? During the last twenty-five years, as people became busier and gyms sprouted up all over the country in response to our limited schedules, workouts were promoted as the best way to lose weight and get in shape in just thirty to sixty minutes.

This isn't to say that gyms, fitness programs or home equipment are the problem either. They aren't. The problem is our perspective that they represent the only or best options for getting exercise. As a society, we have narrowed the scope of what constitutes exercise and the best way to get fit and burn calories. What if these options were part of a much broader view of what you can do for exercise? The good news is that they are, and this broader view is called being active.

Being active opens the definition of exercising to include any activity that gets your heart rate up for a while. If you love the outdoors, you can garden, walk, Nordic walk, bike, hike, row, kayak, cross-country ski, snow shoe or do anything else that you enjoy. If you prefer being with people, you can choose dancing, aerobic classes, team sports or even tennis. Solitary choices can be home exercise videos, interactive exercise games, Pilates, yoga or using the hula hoop, among others. Now you have lots to choose from, and you can define what being active means to you and stay active at a pace and place that fits your lifestyle.

Putting Yourself Last

A forth culprit is letting obligations and schedules define what gets your time and what matters. As more is expected of you at work, at home or in the community, the first thing to go is often what you need or want to do for yourself. The work-home-life balancing act ends up squeezing life out of the equation for so many of us. Despite all the time-saving devices around us, we no longer have extra hours to grocery shop, prepare healthy meals, eat as a family, leisurely socialize with others after dinner or relax on weekends. Instead most of us feel we are racing from one thing to the next, hardly able to catch a breath before getting to the next thing. Yet we are responsible for creating this busyness, even if it doesn't seem that way.

By letting our calendars run our lives or our commitments run our schedules, we may believe we don't have control of them. But the truth is we do control them and can make time for taking care of ourselves, if we think it is important enough. Furthermore, we often take on more tasks with the belief that we are supposed to sacrifice ourselves for our families or careers. And others around us encourage this belief. I'll never forget what a young mother said when she first took one of my workshops. She told the group, "If I don't sacrifice and put myself last, I won't be a good mother." I'm happy to say she feels the opposite today after discovering that by putting herself first and taking care of her health and her needs, her family is much happier and better off.

As host of the healthy lifestyle talk radio show *Living Your Personal Best* for a number of years, I've talked with many guests who didn't see they were putting themselves last until something happened that got their attention. One guest, Mary, was on the fast track in an exciting career, and she loved the adrenaline of her work and the promotions that propelled her up the ladder. She was a type A personality and wanted to succeed at everything, including her marriage. In her early thirties, she felt like she was falling apart and her body was shutting down. She'd had signs something was wrong, such as when she forgot to bring her dress pants to work and had to wear her fitness clothes to a string of important meetings. Then for six months, she thought she had a bad flu or cold that wouldn't go away, until she learned her sickness was more serious than that. Her immune system had been compromised by her stressful lifestyle, and she had to make significant changes to restore her health. When she looks back, she thanks God that her body warned her so early in her life. Now she has a balanced, fulfilling lifestyle that allows her to put herself first.

Another guest, Debra, was in graduate school and taking a full class load and teaching just as many classes. She didn't initially understand why she felt so depressed and lethargic. She didn't want to eat and began feeling sorry for herself, believing she had no control over her choices. As she spiraled further into depression, she became immobilized. It was an insight from her studies that helped her see that she needed to start moving physically to regain her energy, improve her emotional state and regain control of her life. She learned the importance of body-mind integration and taking responsibility for her health.

The one thing that surprises nearly everyone who finally gets it and starts putting themselves first is how well things actually turn out, and not just for themselves. They discover their families are happier because they are happier. They find they have more energy, so they are more productive and effective at work. They learn that cooking meals and having dinner with their kids inspires more communication and being active as a family improves how everyone feels. Time and again, those who give up trying to do everything and slow down to be more connected with themselves discover the opposite of what they imagined is true. They will tell you they are grateful for the lesson and new lease on life.

Relying on Willpower

Another culprit to succeeding at getting fit, that may surprise you, is placing too great an emphasis on mind over matter. Who doesn't think the real barrier to losing weight or getting back into shape is lack of willpower? How often do you judge yourself or someone else for lack of willpower when putting on the pounds, pigging out or going for an extra helping of dessert? Guess what — that isn't the issue! Focusing on willpower as a way of forcing yourself to be good creates the opposite effect and leads to being even more out of control.

The more you exert force, or your will, to make yourself do something, the more you will resist. We all resent being told what to do or feeling pressured. When we are given orders to comply with a program, diet or rule, we rebel. Sure, we may follow the rules for a while to look good or avoid being penalized, but it isn't long before we give up and go back to our old way of doing things. Haven't you done this?

Unfortunately, few people understand how the use of force backfires and instead places blame on those who fail to change their ways. Worse yet, the ones being judged are even harder on themselves. Once you see yourself as a hopeless failure or not strong enough to be good, it becomes harder to try in the future. It is a vicious cycle that often ends in self-criticism and despondency. Even sadder is the belief anyone deserves this, much less you.

We are conditioned in our culture, from childhood into adulthood, to accept enforcement and judgment to get us to behave, so this is familiar and expected. Some people even seek people, such as a boot camp leader or a personal trainer, who will force them to comply with what they know they should do because they think that will keep them in line. They even accept or want harsh admonishment and public humiliation when they don't do as they are told, believing this will work and is what they deserve.

One of my clients, Dorothy, kept asking me when we first started working together what I was going to do to force her to meet her goals. She felt she should be punished for bad behavior and that if I was hard on her, she would have an easier time complying with her agreements. No one deserves this. Furthermore, I explained to her it isn't effective. More often than not, the end result is a withdrawal from trying again in the future. I've had other clients ask me if I was going to get mad at them or do something to make them be good, assuming they've been bad and need to be reprimanded. When I respond by asking them how it would help if I did get angry or try to exert pressure on them, they often admit that my reaction might get them to follow through for a while, but they'd soon be avoiding their goals and our sessions. Force wouldn't help them to change their behaviors, and that is why I don't apply it.

The secret is to stop forcing, bullying, blaming and judging. The method for successfully following through on your goals isn't achieved by willing yourself to behave. It is achieved by choosing activities and foods that are so enjoyable to you physically and emotionally that you willingly select them. Making healthy choices that feel good to you becomes easier when you want more for yourself, feel you deserve better and determine what is best and most enjoyable. Everyone is different in what they find enjoyable and overbearing. You have to know enough about yourself to determine what feels best. For the people who really like and thrive at boot camps, this is a great choice for them.

Once you are motivated for yourself and don't feel threatened by the changes you want to make, your will can be an ally. You can will yourself to get off the couch because you know you will feel better if you go for a short walk. You can will yourself to pay attention to your hunger levels and honor them because then you will be addressing your own needs. You can encourage yourself to prepare meals ahead of time because you know how much easier it will make your week. And instead of fighting it, you will naturally begin to want to do this because it feels good. You won't need your will to help you maintain your new healthy habits, and you won't have your inner rebel trying to throw you off course.

Living in the All or Nothing

One of the most damaging culprits of poor weight loss success — and it is inherent in diets, fitness programs, dietician plans and doctors' orders — is the requirement that you comply fully with the rules and provide proof that you are doing everything exactly as you were told. If you are like most, you do the best you can for a while, and you may even get complimented for following through perfectly. Inevitably, however, you find it harder to follow the guidelines, write everything down and do everything expected of you. When you stop fully complying with the expectations, you probably dread the next appointment, knowing you will get a lecture and a request to do better. And you probably try, yet it often gets harder and harder to comply perfectly.

Well, guess what? No one is perfect. It shouldn't be expected that any of us will ever be able to fully comply with a rigid set of rules. But since it is expected and we can't be perfect, we typically feel guilty and eventually figure what's the use and quit trying at all. We live in an all-or-nothing, good-or-bad, black-or-white culture in which we aren't given room to succeed in the grey zone. That's a problem. Life experiences and choices happen in the grey zone. Situations and events get in the way of perfection, and that doesn't make us bad, lazy or incapable. It makes us human.

Furthermore, by getting caught up in trying to be perfect, we forget what truly matters. When I ask clients to use a food discovery journal, I always get a negative reaction. I expect this because anyone who has filled one out before has done it to demonstrate their compliance with specific nutritional rules and calorie guidelines. But you can use a food journal in a whole new way without rigid rules that is very enlightening and focuses your attention on what is driving your behaviors around food, which is really the issue.

Imagine using a food journal and not having to comply with specific rules. You can use it instead as a discovery tool for how you feel when you eat and what triggers you to overeat or to eat when you aren't hungry. What if you can miss days, create your own format or choose not to write down what you ate — much less measure your foods or count your calories? You can, and you will still gain a lot of insight and information about your eating patterns. I'll explain more about the discovery journal in part 3.

The best approach when creating healthier habits is to build flexibility into the guidelines, allow yourself to make choices that work best in your situation and accept that good is good enough. Good enough is worthy of acknowledgment and applause. With each success, you will likely feel motivated to keep up what you are accomplishing, and you will have a sense of pride that you can really make positive changes.

Believing It Can Wait

Another culprit of unhealthy practices is one you probably know well. It is procrastination. When you are sitting on the sofa watching TV and eating junk food or rushing about doing all the things on your to-do list, it is easy to push away that little voice that says, "I should go for a walk, make a decent dinner or take a soothing bath." Instead you think, "That can wait" or "I'll do that some other time." Your parental voice encourages you to get back on track when you've stopped exercising or eating better, but that other part of you will say "Not today; I'll start tomorrow." And you keep putting off all the things that your body and spirit encourage you to do, believing it can wait. The next thing you know, weeks, months or even years have gone by and you are still putting off making changes.

Part of what is keeping you stuck is the nagging of your parental voice, which you naturally resist. Yet the other voice that resists comes from your belief that exercise and eating healthier really can wait and that another day doesn't matter. While you are right another day doesn't matter, the problem is that people seldom wait just another day. As you continue to put off making changes in your routine, your cholesterol levels, blood pressure and blood sugar levels could well be getting into the danger zones and putting you at risk for disease. Or you could be running yourself into the wall, only to find that out when you can't get up off the floor one day.

The truth is taking better care of your body can't wait. You are putting your health and the lifestyle you take for granted in danger, and you are taking a huge risk in pretending it doesn't matter — possibly more than you fully realize. It isn't just diabetes, heart disease and cancer that can affect you. People who get multiple sclerosis, Lou Gehrig's disease and many other life-altering diseases are increasingly convinced that their unhealthy lifestyles were a cause of their current conditions. I believe I suffered from chronic fatigue because of how I lived my life. Whether our suppositions prove to be true or not, there is no doubt that living in a way that compromises your immune system can be the straw that breaks the camel's back, making it more likely you will contract whatever illness for which you are genetically predisposed. This is why health screenings are so helpful: you can see for yourself what could happen if you don't take action and think instead that a lifestyle change can wait.

Redefining Fitness as a Way of Living

If you haven't had or been around someone with a fit lifestyle, it can be hard to imagine what it really entails or looks like. If you were to ask a hundred people who were living in a fit and healthy way, each would describe their own lifestyle differently, and none of the lifestyles would seem to be the same. As confusing as that might be, the differences are healthy in themselves because they allow for individuality and long-term success. Think about it. No two people like all the same foods or enjoy all the same activities, so why would people have similar healthy habits given the chance to create a lifestyle they could enjoy and easily maintain?

What defines a fit lifestyle best is that it's a way of living and not a fitness program, plan, diet or resolution with a start and stop date. This is a huge shift in thinking from what we've been taught during the twentieth century. Dieting has been popular since the 1920s, and few women have escaped trying them at some point in their lives. The concept of getting into shape since the 1970s has been to reach a target weight, achieved through hard work and uncompromising dedication to specific guidelines, not the creation of healthier habits. For Irene, one of my clients, this distinction was a revelation to her. She said during one of our sessions, "I'm finally getting it, and it is so much easier than I thought. I always thought exercising and dieting was temporary and that I was either going to be on or off them, but that's a trap. I now have more control and feel less panicked because I have a different perspective."

Approaching Fitness Differently

A fit and healthy lifestyle starts with a change in thinking where the emphasis is on the long-term and allows for the ups and downs and disruptions of real life. Real life is unpredictable and makes perfection impossible, so fitness and healthy living exists in that grey zone, not in the black-and-white of good and bad found in programs emphasizing full compliance. In addition, long-term fitness is achieved through moderation, forgiveness and patience instead of all-out intensity, force or striving for quick results. It requires a completely different mindset, which can be challenging to fully grasp after years of pursuing fitness and dieting to reach a goal.

Living a fit lifestyle also shifts the emphasis from what others think is right for you to what you think is right for yourself. This shift may seem intimidating at first because you may not know how or where to begin. But you will soon learn that you do know where to begin because you know what you do and don't like and you know what does and doesn't feel good. You may be thinking, "Oh, I already know what I'm supposed to do; I just don't do it," but what will surprise you is that most of that "knowledge" is probably not right. There is a reason you aren't able to get started; therefore, what you think you need to do isn't really what you are supposed to do. I know I am turning conventional wisdom on its head but trust I will show you the way.

Having said that, I will also say a fit and healthy lifestyle includes eating healthier foods, being active, getting enough sleep and water, reducing stress, taking a multivitamin and limiting alcohol. This, no doubt, is what you would say you know. What you probably don't know is how to put these habits successfully into practice as part of your daily lifestyle. You don't really know *how* to live healthier in a way that works for you.

You may wonder if you will ever be able to make this shift in thinking about your lifestyle, and that's to be expected. This approach is very different, and you will ease into it on your own terms and at your own pace the more you learn and experience it. In the meantime, be open-minded to the process, and you may discover it grows on you and is just the solution you've been waiting for.

Getting That Great Feeling

There is nothing better than feeling absolutely wonderful. When asked by a clerk, "How are you?" a woman in front of me at a coffee shop once said, "Absolutely wonderful!" She clearly meant it. She was smiling and relaxed, and she had that spring in her step that said she was indeed having a super day and felt great about herself. Wow! How often do you hear that or feel that for yourself? Even I felt a twinge of jealously as I realized I didn't happen to feel absolutely wonderful that morning, and I wanted to experience that. Who doesn't want to feel that good inside and out?

Unfortunately for so many people, feeling great seems far outside the realm of their reality. Life just isn't like that and hasn't been like that for years. Think back to a time when you felt invincible, confident, energetic and able to do anything. When was the last time you felt really great physically and mentally? If it has been way too long or you can't even think of a time, don't despair. It is still possible to feel this. If hasn't been that long, relive the feelings. By bringing them back into your reality, they will be powerful motivators to keep your healthy lifestyle on track.

Those that succeed in creating a fit way of living discover to their delight that it feels really good. They had no idea it could be so wonderful to have greater energy, stamina, strength, fitness and health. And once they tasted the freedom that comes from being able to do most anything and feeling good about themselves, they were motivated to keep up their new routines and to do even more for themselves.

The transformation is like finding precious gems after chiseling through hard rock. You get hooked and want more of those beauties. The transformation can even lead to a love for chiseling other types of rock to create a work of art. Who knows where the process will take you? There are thousands of people, myself included, who discovered an unexpected passion for fitness after creating a realistic and enjoyable fitness routine that became part of their lives.

Doing It for You

Doing something for yourself is totally different than doing it for someone else. When you do something for another person, you often feel you should do it because you don't want to let them down. Making lifestyle changes for someone else can backfire, though, because you will come to resist the changes and the person requesting them. However, if you are at the point where you are willing to make the change and see the benefits, then having someone else to hold you accountable will really help.

The toughest part of creating a healthy and fit lifestyle is getting started and sticking with it. A new lifestyle takes longer to fully adopt than simply creating one small new habit, because there are so many aspects to what you do throughout the day tied to your health and fitness. You may be ready to make the changes and be willing to do anything, yet the reality is you can only change so much at a time. Other people don't know what is realistic for you and may suggest too many changes at once and expect too much, and soon you may pressure yourself to comply with their wishes and feeling resentful.

It matters what role you and others decide to play in your lifestyle changes. If you let those around you tell you what you should do, you will struggle to succeed on your own terms, and you will almost assuredly fail to meet their standards. On the other hand, if you set clear boundaries and make it clear you know what you are doing and are only interested in having someone's support under certain conditions, then you will give yourself the right to start off slowly and discover what works best for you to reach your longer-term vision.

Needing accountability to succeed isn't a character flaw or indicative of how successful you can eventually be. It is being honest that creating and maintaining changes — even small ones — are tough, and that without accountability, you can easily slide back into what is more familiar and comfortable. Picking the right person to account to for your actions can make or break your ability to succeed. If you choose someone who judges you harshly when you don't follow through, you will feel pressured to perform and tempted to lie. Soon you will give up, believing you can't meet the person's expectations and can't succeed. But if you have someone who never judges you but is there instead to be witness, helping you examine what works and what doesn't, and celebrate your successes, then you have a support system to keep you going.

In time, you will have a eureka moment, as my mother had after a couple of years of working with me. She realized she was exercising for herself because she wanted to. "I am no longer doing this for you," she proudly said during one of our calls. "I am now doing it for me." I was so excited for her. She no longer needed me to hold her accountable, which had made such a difference in helping her get started and stay on track up to that point. When she turned the corner, she could recognize the antsy feeling when she wasn't moving enough, and she really wanted to get out for a walk or go to the gym she enjoyed. She also valued how good she felt and how far she had come, and she didn't want to lose that sense of well-being and accomplishment.

Are You Ready to Change Your Mindset?

There is no point trying to adopt lifestyle changes if you aren't really ready, as I've said before, because all you will do is *try* instead of *commit*. Trying leads to frustration, disappointment in yourself and the determination you just can't really do it. It takes a commitment to succeed even if you've learned a process that makes the change easier.

Very often what keeps you from being ready is what you believe and feel from past experiences. You may not believe the payoff is worth the effort until the price becomes too high to stay where you are. When you have that defining moment, don't let it pass you by. That is the time to take action.

Getting Resolved

For many of us, a commitment to fitness and a healthy lifestyle comes when something happens that we can't ignore. There comes a moment when you are either humiliated enough, scared enough or frustrated enough to have a defining moment where you resolve to change immediately. The defining moment can happen in an instant.

My defining moment came when I was standing in front of my mirror after putting on five dress sizes in just fifteen months and recovering from yet another three-month round of being bedridden with chronic fatigue. What came to mind was if I didn't change my ways, I might never feel or look better. I thought if I didn't act soon, it may become too late to do anything about it. That was a wake-up call I couldn't ignore, and I didn't. Nearly everyone with a fitness or healthy-lifestyle success story had a pivotal moment that led to a resolve to make a lifestyle change.

What these people will also most likely tell you is that the wake-up call that got them to respond wasn't the first one they experienced. Before we act, there is often a series of experiences that have the potential to be the one event that changes our perspective. It is the accumulation of these experiences that gives you the feeling you are being hit over the head by a two-by-four when the next event comes along. The resolve to take action is also a matter of letting the last event become the defining moment that changes your behavior and motivates you to overcome your numbness and inertia. This moment is what propels you to make healthy lifestyle changes that are hard to make without a catalyst. For Brittany, the defining moment was the diagnosis of skin cancer; Nick's was testicular cancer. Elizabeth's wake-up call was not being able to keep up with her kids; Charise's was taking a diabetes survey in a magazine and seeing she was at high risk; Theresa's was the photo of herself at a wedding.

If you don't take action when you have this experience, whatever resolve you have will slip away. The moment can leave nearly as quickly as it came, so when it does happen, keep it by taking some action. Taking action doesn't have to be a big step. Anything that moves you out of inaction will help you hold onto that fragile resolve. With each step you take, you build momentum and create new thoughts and behaviors that solidify changes in your life.

Even if you don't have that defining moment, you can use this book or this paragraph in its place. You can look back at missed opportunities and realize that today is the day to take a small step toward changing the way you take care of yourself. And that first little step, starting with a decision and doing one thing to put yourself in action — like taking a short walk — will start the ball rolling as if you had experienced a major wake-up call.

Taking Stock

What you will likely discover when you have a wake-up call is just how out of balance you've been and how much more you want for yourself. You may find out that you've been suffering in many ways, and you just didn't notice it before. Suffering is more than a physical or emotional experience; it is also mental and spiritual. The more we suffer, the more we pull away from experiencing how much it hurts, and when you stop feeling the pain, you also stop feeling anything else. You either feel or you don't feel, and the less you feel, the more disconnected you become from yourself and what matters to you. This is how you shift into denial about how overweight, sick, uncomfortable, unhappy or scared you are.

The real problem that keeps many people from living a healthier life is what they believe about themselves and how they've repressed their emotions. Their undermining beliefs and repressed emotions are the baggage they carry around, whether they realize it or not. It is our beliefs and feelings that drive our behaviors. So any baggage about your body, self-image, food or activity will prevent you from doing the things you claim you want to do for yourself, such as having more work-life-health balance, choosing healthy options or following your heart and dreams.

If you have a lot of mental or emotional baggage, you may drive yourself into the ground by overdoing, attempting to reach unattainable goals, beating yourself up, feeling unworthy and shutting down. This was my story. On the outside, you may look and function as if everything is fine, but it isn't. And until a crisis occurs, you may not even know something's wrong. You will live in denial. Worse, if you don't feel good about yourself, you probably won't be willing to put effort into changing. I had a client once who stopped seeing me after a few weeks, claiming she didn't feel she deserved to be good to herself. She wasn't able to stick around long enough to let the process help her change that perspective. She needed to go through her own healing first, so I wished her well, knowing she had to follow her own inner guidance.

Taking stock is an opportunity to consciously check in with yourself to uncover how you really feel and what your heart and soul are telling you. This doesn't happen in a day, but it can start then. To fully uncover what is inside can take months or even years, and it can often involve journaling, help from various types of practitioners or healers and spiritual introspection. Discovery journaling, which I mentioned earlier and is introduced later in this book, is one tool you can use to gain insight into and release some of the baggage.

Loving Yourself

If you have come to believe you are unable to follow through, guilty for not getting it right, bad at dieting or fitness programs, too fat to be loved or even unworthy of doing what it takes to change, understand that this isn't the real you talking. This is only what you have come to believe and feel is true because of past experiences, what others have told you and unrealistic expectations. This doesn't negate your feelings, which are real and which you have a right to express. Instead negative feelings about yourself indicate the need to release self-critical beliefs and create new ones aligned with who you really are. We are all capable of succeeding. We are not what we look like, and we are all worth the effort, no matter what others might have said or you have subsequently told yourself.

If you were to ask your friends and family what they love most about you, you will probably hear that you have many qualities that they cherish and wish you could see in yourself. Try it. Ask people close to you what five things they love or really like about you and write them down. Accept what your loved ones are saying, and appreciate that you really are special, capable and gifted. Now ask yourself what five things you love about yourself and really listen. You may be surprised by how many things make you special and what you learn about why you deserve to love yourself even more than you do.

Instead of focusing on what you don't like about yourself, you can focus on all the things that are positive. The more you remind yourself of why you make a difference and what makes you loved by others, the easier it is to feel more love for yourself. At first it may seem as if the positive qualities are about someone other than you, so to bring these qualities closer to home, think of yourself as a child or young adult with all these characteristics. You have always been uniquely and wonderfully you, and through a younger set of eyes, you may be able to feel how true this is. The more you love yourself, the more you will respect and want to do what is best for you. When this happens, you will be open to taking better care of yourself physically, emotionally and spiritually.

Breaking Free

Change requires enough optimism, determination and desire to break free of feeling indifferent and ambivalent. When you feel hopeless or stuck, it is hard to muster any interest in taking action or making a change. And it doesn't take much to become resigned and feel hopeless after being stressed or temporarily derailed from making progress, experiencing repeated failures or getting depressed. Once despondent it can take considerable effort to overcome inertia and take the first step toward action.

What gives you the extra strength needed to break free is the hope that this time will be different. You have probably tried everything you thought would work, and you may question if this book or anything else out there will really work for you. That is understandable. You have probably been through a lot, judged for not doing enough and convinced that you are destined to be the way you are. Only with hope that there really is a better way than what you've already tried will you give it your all one more time.

When Maria came to me, she was very concerned about her health and had reached a point where she knew it was critical to do something about it. She didn't have the stamina she needed to support her speaking and travel schedule, and she noticed that during the past six months she hadn't been feeling at that well. She was at risk for heart disease because of her weight, and she knew in her heart that she had to take better care of herself. But she couldn't get herself to go to the gym where she had a membership, nor could she avoid the carbohydrates she loved or make time to eat when she needed food. Instead, she let her health slide and looked the other way. She felt helpless in her ability to stick with better behaviors and struggled within herself over what to do. She held out hope I could teach her a better way to take back control of her lifestyle and break free from her unhealthy behaviors.

There is one other thing that will help you break free: believing you have the right to set boundaries, be treated with respect and be given an emotionally safe environment to put your toes back in the water. Without this, you could find yourself overwhelmed, pushed too far and giving up. You know yourself and your feelings better than anyone else does. You know what is realistic for you, what you can really do and what you need. Now is the time to stand up for yourself and to set limits that best serve you without concern for what anyone else thinks is right.

Part Two

A New Way of Thinking
about Eating, Exercise & Self-Care

The 3 Cs for Regaining Confidence and Control

A New Way of Thinking about Eating, Exercise & Self-Care

The 3 Cs for Regaining Confidence and Control

In this section you will be introduced to a new way of relating to food, fitness and well-being that will allow you to regain pleasure in eating, activity and making yourself a priority. What I will share with you is the secret to making healthy and fit choices, and the secret isn't radical or complicated. Instead, it is surprisingly simple, obvious, freeing and eye-opening. Even better, it will help you find your own path to regaining health, happiness and well-being that is enjoyable and easy to follow, instead of restrictive and unpleasant.

The secret is found in what I call the 3 Cs: consciousness, clarity and choices. These concepts will give you confidence that you can be in control and make the best choices for yourself when it comes to food, activities, and how you feel. They will also help you stay motivated and on track in your journey of living a healthier and happier life.

You've been taught a lot about eating, exercise and healthcare, but the one thing you haven't been taught is the thing that will give you the confidence and control to succeed. That one thing is how to govern your emotional and mental mindset, or how you think and feel about things. Your mindset, tucked away in your subconscious, drives your attitude toward and behaviors around taking care of yourself and making healthier choices.

Sue discovered her own mindset when she came to understand what was getting in the way of meeting her exercise goals. She said, "The problem is between my ears, and what I feed my mind." She observed how she'd been resisting her exercise routine, and as she observed where the resistance was coming from, she saw it was stemming from her beliefs about herself, exercise and her age. When she changed her beliefs, she changed her thinking and overcame the resistance.

What changed her mind was having insight into her beliefs and recognizing she could think differently. You can do the same. I'm going to show you a new way to look at your own experiences and see them in a new light so you can feel inspired and motivated to make healthier choices and stick with them.

You will learn how to work with what is going on inside your head by addressing old patterns, limiting beliefs and negative thoughts that don't support you, and then creating new beliefs and strategies that will help you succeed. It is a process of working from the inside out instead of being told what to do from the outside in. The 3 Cs give you the tools needed to change your behaviors through self-awareness, self-reflection, ah-ha insights, positive thinking, affirming beliefs and self-motivating choices.

Consciousness without Judgment

You can't change the way you do things or make different choices about your habits if you aren't conscious of what you are doing in the first place. For example, if you are overeating but not paying attention, you won't be aware enough of how you really feel to stop eating. You will subconsciously keep on chewing away.

Think about it. How often do you overeat to the point of being horribly full? Do you then wonder why you couldn't stop — or worse, do you beat yourself up because you didn't stop? Do you even know what being full or overly full feels like? Most people overeat regularly, believing that is just the way it is for them, and they don't register how uncomfortable being full really makes them feel. We tune out surprisingly well what we don't want to process, feel or deal with.

I remember when my client Brandy discovered just how awful being full really felt. She overate most nights of the week, usually ending up on the couch asleep. She didn't even think about it. It is just what she did, and the part she struggled with the most was waking up around two in the morning and making her way groggily upstairs to bed. As we began to work together, she started to pay attention to how she felt physically when she ate, and she observed that she started off eating to feel better but ended up feeling sick. She didn't like how horrible it felt, and she was amazed she hadn't really noticed this before. The feeling was so unpleasant to her that she found it easy to stop overeating after that. Now, years later, she still avoids overeating.

We also tune things out about our activity and lifestyle habits, where doing something unhealthy is often just a subconscious behavior. If you end up watching TV, doing chores or working instead of exercising or preparing healthy meals, you are subconsciously choosing to avoid a healthier behavior. You may make these choices out of habit or avoidance even though you know you will feel badly about it later. You may even feel the choice is outside of your control.

This is how Penny felt when she called me looking for help to get back into shape. She had not been focused on fitness since her son was born nearly five years before, and she didn't see anyway she could fit exercise into her schedule. She worked all day, and when she got home, she didn't feel she could leave again to go to the gym without feeling guilty or upsetting her kids.

In our discussions we focused on exploring her options. She talked to her husband about ways she could make time for herself, which he was eager to help her do. She realized that she felt guilty about taking any time away from her kids, and that was holding her back. She also explored ways to involve the kids in activities on the weekends, as well as ways she could leave work fifteen minutes early and arrive home fifteen minutes later to fit something in after work. The new strategy seemed doable.

In Brittany's case, she found dealing with her kids easier when they watched TV. In the evenings, the whole family would eat dinner while watching their favorite shows. They would start off with the main course and then bring in various desserts or popcorn until the kids had to go off and do their homework. Then she and her husband would finish off what was left. Brittany had no idea how much food she was eating while in front of the TV, but she did know it didn't feel very good. Breaking this habit wasn't easy. She decided to have the family eat at the dinner table, and what surprised her was how willing the kids were to make the change and have a chance to talk about school. It was she and her husband that felt pulled back to the TV, and that, she finally understood, was because in the TV room, they could hide from the problems in their marriage.

By tuning out and avoiding feelings, you can't be mindful of the choices you are making and of their consequences. Instead, you have excuses about why you couldn't have made the choices, such as working long hours and too many commitments, or because you have a family or are a single parent. Those reasons aren't what really keep you from finding time to take care of yourself. What is keeping you from finding time is choosing to make other choices without fully realizing it and often saying yes to things that you later wish you could have said no to.

Saying no was hard for my client Abigail, who had been struggling with her priorities. She often found herself saying yes to people at work or where she volunteered, which took time away from what really mattered to her: her family, health and spiritual well-being. As we talked about this, she began to see a connection between wanting to please others and how she had tried to please her father, who had not paid attention to her and had left her wanting acknowledgment and appreciation. She had never made the connection before, and once she understood it, she found it easier to say no to things that didn't matter enough. By becoming conscious of what was driving her to say yes, she no longer had to beat herself up for taking on too much, and she found her voice to say no much more easily.

It is hard to be conscious of what you don't want to see or own up to, as these things are usually accompanied by painful emotions and judgment at the hands of your inner critic. We are so self-critical that to avoid the guilt and shame, we often look the other way. When you harshly judge your behaviors, you often won't want to face them, and this leads to living less consciously and more in denial at your own expense.

Seeing Behaviors through a New Lens

Most of us have been taught to believe that our behaviors define us and that what you do is who you are. If you eat a dozen brownies, you did a bad thing, and you are bad by default. This has been further drummed into our heads by how we talk to ourselves and one another about our behaviors toward food and fitness. How often have you said to yourself or to someone else, "I was bad yesterday. I didn't work out, I didn't stick to my diet, I didn't do as much or as little as I said I would. I am so bad. I can't be good. I don't know if I can do this," or something similar?

Clients are always quick to tell me at the start of a session, "I was so bad last week because …" or "I failed to do what I was supposed to." They weren't bad. They didn't fail. Nor does it make sense to judge your behavior as good or bad. That doesn't serve you, help you or change anything. Think about it: even if you say you did something bad or you are bad, you probably still do it. It doesn't change your behavior to focus on it or reinforce it. In fact, you will probably do what was "bad" even more just to prove yourself right. You will be as bad or as incapable of following through as you tell yourself you are.

Rather than focusing on whether your behavior was right or wrong, good or bad, it is better to have an understanding of what drove you to have that behavior in the first place. There can be any number of reasons, many of which you don't control. What you can't control are the curve balls thrown at you during the day, such as emergencies, other people's plans and getting ill. What you can control are your choices, but to make better choices, sometimes you need better information, more awareness of the situation you are in and the knowledge of why you feel driven to make the choices you do.

For example, there can be many different explanations for overeating. Here are eight possible reasons:

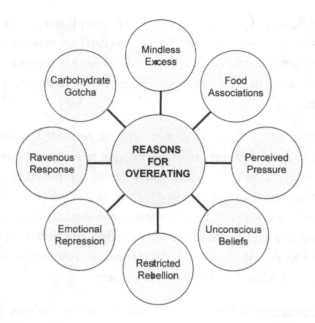

- <u>A Ravenous Response</u>: If you wait to eat until you are ravenous, you will inevitably overeat. You will feel like you can't stop yourself because physiologically and psychologically you are driven to make up for the lack of food earlier in the day or the meal you skipped a few hours ago.

- <u>The Carbohydrate Gotcha</u>: If you only eat carbohydrates — particularly simple carbohydrates, such as pastries or white bread, which are digested very quickly — for your meal or snack, you won't realize you've overdone it until you have eaten way too much.

- <u>Mindless Excess</u>: If you are focused on something like a TV show, a book, work or a conversation when you eat, you won't be aware of when you get full.

- <u>Food Associations</u>: If you tend to eat when you aren't hungry or eat too much when you get home from work, celebrate great news, complete a difficult project or feel sick, for example, you may be eating because you associate food with similar situations from your past.

- <u>Perceived Pressure</u>: If you think you have to eat or to continue eating because others are eating, food is presented to you, your spouse is still eating or everyone else is having dessert, then you may be allowing other people to have power over your decisions.

- <u>Subconscious Beliefs</u>: If you eat everything on your plate as you were told to do, always have dessert after dinner, feel you can't get enough, eat more food than you want because it is readily available or it might be thrown away, you are applying subconscious beliefs about food you probably grew up with.

- <u>Restricted Rebellion</u>: If you think you will be restricted from having enough food in the near future or you won't get to have any more of the wonderful food you are eating now, you will feel compelled to eat all of it while you can, even to the point of feeling sick. This is an emotional reaction to believing you will be restricted and deprived. The same thing happens when you have been restricted in the past and didn't get enough, whether that was during childhood or a recent diet. Another term for this is "deprivation backlash," as I mentioned earlier.

- <u>Emotional Repression</u>: If you are feeling upset, sad or anxious, food can be a coping mechanism you will turn to in place of really feeling what is happening. To bury the feelings, you will overeat and use food as a pacifier for your feelings and as a way of getting your needs met quickly. This is called "emotional eating," which is somewhat of a misnomer because it is really repression eating.

With this new understanding about what might be driving you to overeat, you may have immediate insights about your behaviors. But the choices you make aren't as obvious as you might think. We are all complicated, and what is really driving your behavior may not be what you initially believe, or your initial insight may be just the tip of the iceberg. The reason could also be a mix of things: it could first appear as a ravenous response that is masking a subconscious belief and a restrictive rebellion pattern.

I've found that many people believe they have emotional eating issues, and very often they do. But just as often, they are confusing emotional eating with other causes, which limits their ability to see what else may the source of their eating behaviors. I've also worked with people who weren't dealing with emotional eating issues at all, and it would have been a disservice to start off looking for them.

Instead of jumping to conclusions and assumptions about your behaviors, become curious about them as if you are a neutral observer without any reason for judgment. Notice times when you are still eating despite feeling full and think, "Isn't that interesting." Also pay attention when you reach for food if you aren't hungry and consider if there is a reason for that. Notice I didn't say a bad reason. What is driving your behaviors has nothing to do with being good or bad. These drivers are simply things to recognize and understand as you gain greater clarity.

For Gail, letting go of judgment was hard to do. She felt so guilty whenever she overate and was quick to tell me how bad she had been. I would remind her that what mattered wasn't that her behavior was bad but instead what was driving her to keep eating. Instead of judging herself, I asked her to be curious and get in touch with what she was thinking or feeling before and during eating, or even afterward if she couldn't be mindful sooner. She was being triggered to eat and needed to understand why.

This also applies to other behaviors that aren't healthy or best for you. Be mindful when you skip a walk or decide not to go to the gym and take note — without making yourself wrong. Be aware when you end the day and haven't had much water or have drunk lots of alcohol. Take another look when you are getting agitated, snapping at people or pushing yourself to the limit. Think, okay, that happened, and there is a reason behind it worth understanding. With that understanding, you can begin to make small changes that will help you behave in a way that honors you and your body.

Ending the Judgment

Judgment is a reflection of what you believe to be true about yourself. When we judge ourselves, we are repeating the negative self-talk and beliefs that devalue our worth. Judgment affects your self-esteem and often creates feelings that are hard to face, which can lead to emotional eating, stress and depression.

Feeling judged is painful, no matter if it is ourselves or someone else that inspires us to feel that way. This is why judgment makes it so hard to be objective. You can't be neutral and curious if you feel judged, guilty or shamed. When you feel that way, all you want to do is look the other way and avoid the source of criticism.

We don't only judge ourselves harshly; we also target others. But what you may not realize is when you judge others, you actually judge yourself. Have you ever seen an overweight person getting a double order of french fries or something else you think isn't healthy? Did you then think, "Look at that fatso. She shouldn't be doing that. Doesn't she know better?" Then consider this: if she doesn't care what you think, then she doesn't take on your judgment. Instead you are the one being affected, and that judgment of the other person becomes a reflection of your own self-judgment. Perhaps you aren't in the best shape either, and what you are ordering isn't always so healthy. None of us is perfect, and we tend to harshly judge in others the things we don't like or feel good about in ourselves.

Judgment is like pointing a finger at someone and having three of your fingers pointing back at you. As you judge someone, the words and feelings are also reflected back at you.

Now, if you turn this around and believe someone is judging you: you can only be affected if you allow yourself to feel judged and take that judgment on. By taking it on, you assume the harsh judgment you have about yourself is validated. You may even assume someone is judging you who isn't, by interpreting their look or behavior as having something to do with you, your weight or your choices.

Misinterpreted self-judgment is what happened to Diana, who had assumed in high school that she wasn't liked because she was fat. It was the story she carried around with her. If someone didn't seem to warm up to her, their actions validated how unworthy she was because of her weight. Years later at a class reunion, she found herself talking to one of the guys who had shown no interest in her back in school. She learned she wasn't liked for a totally different reason that had nothing to do with her weight. It was her attitude. She was stunned. She had interpreted everything for years through the lens of being too fat, only to find out it was her shame about her weight that pushed people away.

When you no longer judge yourself, you are released from the shame and can focus on other things. Have you ever noticed how thin people who have overweight friends seem oblivious to their friends' size, or how those who are overweight and proud of it don't treat their weight as an issue? If you love your body and yourself the way you are, you won't focus on size but on enjoying life and those around you. The more you practice non-judgment, the less you judge yourself in all facets of your life.

Granted, non-judgment isn't easy in a culture that promotes ultrathin figures and celebrity perfection. Yet there is a growing number of famous role models who are proud to be who they are and to accept all of themselves, including Oprah, Whoopi Goldberg, Emme, Queen Latifah and Mo'Nique, who launched a line of clothes called Big, Beautiful and Loving It. Less well-known yet just as powerful is Meg Barnhouse, who is a writer, minister and singer-songwriter. Meg is also proud to accept her size and to smash her self-critic and others' ideals of being thin. When Meg was on my radio show, she talked about looking at pictures of herself years younger when she thought she had been too fat and realizing how beautiful she really was. She realized that seeing herself as fat had been coming from her judgmental state of mind.

A good daily practice is to become conscious of your behaviors, and to respond to them by thinking, "Isn't that interesting." As you come to appreciate that your behaviors are not good or bad, you will realize there is always a story behind them and you are doing the best you can. From this perspective, you will have more compassion for yourself and will be open to learning your inner story and seeing what is keeping you from doing something healthier.

What is Your Consciousness Level?

Consciousness Level

Rate how conscious you are of each activity from 0 to 5.
0 = not conscious; 5 = very conscious

<u>0–5</u>

I know when I get hungry.
I eat when I am hungry.
I eat at set times, regardless of how hungry I am.
I know when you start to feel.
I have a hard time stopping my eating even when I am getting full.
I know what being full feels like.

I am aware of my self-talk throughout the day.
I know how often I label myself bad or unworthy.
I have an idea of when or how often I judge myself.
I know what story I am carrying about myself.

I am aware of how much physical activity I have done this week.
I notice how much energy I have during the day.
I am aware of how I physically feel throughout the day.
I know I have a choice about whether I have enough time for fitness.
I know what drives my decisions about exercise.
I notice if I blame myself for less than perfect behavior.

Score 60–80   You have great awareness of your body, behaviors and physical needs.

Score 40–60   You have good awareness of how you feel and what you are doing.

Score 20–40   You have limited awareness of yourself and your behaviors.

As you think about your answers and score, don't judge them. Just think, "Isn't that interesting," and be curious. The less awareness you have, the more you will likely learn about yourself in the pages ahead.

Clarity through Understanding

Once you are conscious of what you are doing without judging it, you can be open to fully investigating and understanding what is triggering behaviors that aren't helping you succeed. This self-awareness is an opportunity to be curious and learn more about yourself and what is driving you to make choices that don't feel good.

Gaining self-awareness is *not* about trying to figure out why you don't do as you should, make bad choices or are not good at something. That kind of thinking is what got you here in the first place. It is time to banish "should," "bad" and "not good at" from your vocabulary. These words distract you from being open to finding out what is really making it hard for you to live the life you really want.

Some of your behaviors will adjust quite easily as you pay more attention to what you are doing and how you feel physically. When many people get in touch with their feeling of fullness, they find they don't want to feel that way anymore. They discover, as Brandy did, that feeling full is too uncomfortable, and they intuitively stop eating before getting to that point. Choosing to eat without distractions, like TV or driving, also makes it easier to stop.

Doreen, another one of my clients, amazed herself and her friends when she visited them for dinner a couple of weeks after she began paying attention to her hunger and fullness. They had Newman's Hint O' Mint cookies for dessert, which Doreen loved and often couldn't stop eating. She had enjoyed the meal, felt satisfied afterward, and when the plate of cookies went around she took one. Her friends each took three, but she wanted to start with just one for a change. She found herself paying more attention to how good the cookie tasted instead of devouring it and missing the experience. When she finished it, she realized that she didn't need another one. She wanted to remain satisfied instead of eating unconsciously and becoming too full.

The following week, Doreen bought one of those gigantic cookies while out walking with a friend. After a few bites, she tossed it in the trash. She found that she really didn't want any more than she had eaten. Her girlfriend was speechless. Doreen was not one to pass up cookies, much less not finish one or, even more shocking, to throw it away. But Doreen felt empowered and done with the cookie.

Becoming conscious is easy. It is harder to address the thoughts, beliefs and feelings you don't realize you are having that drive your behaviors toward food, fitness and taking care of yourself.

Imagine observing that someone is ignoring you. That leads you to think you are being ignored because you are fat, which reinforces how unworthy you feel you are. You will probably feel hurt and ashamed and, to soothe yourself, turn to your favorite comfort foods. When you realize how much you've eaten, you may feel even more guilty and shameful, which will drive you to eat even more, further validating how unlikable and undeserving you really are. This is classic emotional eating, and it demonstrates that your beliefs and feelings are the subconscious drivers of your behavior.

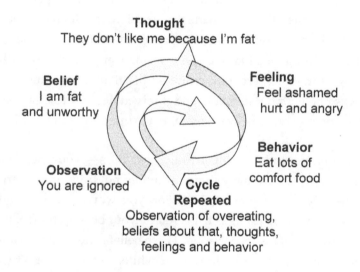

Another example (which is one we've all experienced) happens when you eat too much and think you have blown your diet. This thought validates the belief that you can't control yourself and will never be able to lose weight. You feel hopeless and disgusted, and then you look for something else to eat, which proves your belief right.

This cycle may seem obvious once it is explained, but when it is happening, you often aren't aware of the beliefs or feelings that lead to the overeating (or any other unhealthy behaviors). In the moment, all you know is you can't get enough food, you've eaten too much, you wish you hadn't, and you feel out of control.

What is shocking about this series of events is most of what we observe is filtered by what we choose to see. Our thoughts about our observations are seldom based on actual facts but on our interpretation of events from the past or expectations about the future. Those thoughts then validate the beliefs we learned from our parents, teachers, peers and society, which in turn causes feelings that we don't realize we are having. Those feelings then lead to behaviors we judge as good or bad.

Yet in the moment that we choose to respond with a specific behavior, we are often unaware of any cause but the circumstances we're reacting to, and we usually think we are doing the best we can. And we are. After the moment has passed, however, we attack our behavior and ourselves, forgetting we didn't see any other option when we made a decision or that we made a choice that seemed like the right one at the time.

My client Anita had chosen to clean out her closets and de-clutter her house when she had some time off from work rather than begin exercising. She had been under a lot of stress, and organizing was something that calmed her and helped her transition to being at home for a while. When she made this decision, she did it consciously and told me that this had to be done and was more important to her than exercising. Yet a couple of weeks later, she complained that she wasn't losing weight and was really bad for not getting in enough time for exercise. I reminded her that at the time she chose not to exercise, she was fine with her decision, and it served her best to clean out her closets. To judge that action harshly now was not going to support her in reaching her goals.

It is pointless, damaging and draining to judge behaviors — your own or anyone else's — because they are based on many things you may not fully understand. If you did understand what really caused your behavior, you would have more compassion. Recognize that what you are doing is triggered by your beliefs and feelings, which for most of us lie hidden in the subconscious. These beliefs and feelings cannot easily be labeled right or wrong, good or bad, black or white, just as it doesn't make sense to label your eating, activity or self-care behaviors this way.

Observing Your Behaviors

The only way to stop the cycle is to know when you are behaving in a way that doesn't serve your goals or make you feel good. Since it is hard to be in touch with your beliefs and feelings, the easiest place to start is by becoming aware of what it is you are doing or how you physically feel as a result of your behavior. If you are full yet still eating, being conscious of the full feeling can help you see what you are doing.

Initially you may only be aware of your behaviors hours after you did or didn't do something, but the more you practice being in touch with yourself, the sooner you will notice them. For example, at first you may realize you skipped going for a walk the day afterward because you felt a bit sluggish. The next time you skip your walk, you may realize it the same day and find a way to do something about it that night. And the following time, you may notice just as you are changing your plans and catch yourself in time to go for that walk.

Joellen is an example of someone who was so busy during the day that her behavior choices didn't fully register until she was getting ready for bed. She would overeat at lunch, eat Fritos as she ran out the door to go home from work and mindlessly consume snack foods for dinner while catching up with paperwork or emails. Yet as the weeks went by and we talked more about hunger levels, she started to notice them sooner. She began noticing within an hour of when she overate because she started observing that she didn't feel so well. This insight led her to be more aware as she ate, and this awareness helped her uncover what was driving her food choices.

Kathy had a different experience. She had days when she was highly conscious and other days when she was tuned out. The more she practiced being aware, the easier it got, but if she let her self-awareness slide for too long, then she completely forgot about paying attention.

It takes effort to remind yourself to pay attention, so it helps to have something that supports you in being conscious. Journals or logs are probably the most helpful because they give you a visible reminder and a place to record what you are doing or experiencing. There is no one way to keep a journal, and most people like to come up with their own approach. In part 3, I will introduce you to the hunger scale, discovery journal and fitness journal, which are very helpful in gaining greater awareness.

Getting In Touch with Your Feelings

As you become conscious of your behaviors, you can start to question what is driving them. Feelings are the primary cause of emotional eating, resisting being active and neglecting yourself. Beliefs fuel the intensity of your emotions and affect your reasoning about your eating, exercise and well-being behaviors. Feelings or beliefs or both can impact your behavior. We'll start with feelings.

You may already be in touch with how you feel. If so, you'll be able to recognize when certain feelings cause certain behaviors. We all get annoyed, disappointed, upset, sad and stressed, just for starters, and we have needs that are associated with these feelings that aren't always met, such as a need for respect. One of the reasons these feelings aren't addressed is that we live in a culture where letting feelings be known isn't welcomed, or we are too busy or exhausted to bring them up. A way to soothe the feelings and feel better is to turn to food, alcohol or even drugs for emotional comfort.

That is just what Melanie did when she got overcharged by her contractor. She found herself heading straight to the refrigerator after a call with the customer service manager, who told her she not only had not been overbilled but she was also being charged with a late fee for not paying on time. She was furious as she pulled out pie leftover from the night before and the whipped cream. She calmed down as the food did its magic and decided to pay the bill and accept there was nothing else she could do, but the problem was not fully resolved. Underneath her calm, she was still seething and choosing not to deal with it. And that night, she binged on dessert to the point of almost being sick.

Emotional overeating and drinking commonly occur at night. Feelings most often want to come to the surface at the end of the day when you are finally getting a breather from the demands of work or your family. But if this still isn't a good time to bring up your feelings or you don't have a way to share and address them, then food and drinking is where you may turn. By recognizing your feelings and why you are having them, you can identify what will help you resolve the problem and how you can best get your needs addressed.

My client Roger had lost his brother to heart disease at an early age. This frightened him. His father had also died of a heart attack, and Roger didn't feel his body was functioning as well as it should be in his mid forties. The loss of his brother was also painful because he and his brother had taken over their father's business, and now Roger had to keep it going alone. But he kept up the business, worked out at the gym before work and afterward went home to his wife and kids. Once home, he would have a few drinks, eat dinner around 6:30 and then keep on eating. He couldn't seem to stop, even though he would eventually become uncomfortably full to the point of being almost ill.

What he needed was some time to relieve the tension and stress from the office and get some time to feel replenished and do something for himself that he enjoyed. He loved golf, and he discovered playing some holes of golf or doing some practice shots after work on his way home at a local driving range helped relieve his tension. A half-hour at the range made all the difference, and he would leave feeling refreshed and ready to be with his family. He also started to take twenty minutes after dinner to be by himself or to be with his wife to chat about his day. These changes curbed his drinking and his weeknight overeating.

If you don't find it easy to feel or prefer to keep your feelings to yourself, you may be making your situation worse by avoiding your feelings. Feelings that aren't expressed and released will eventually make themselves known in other ways. One way is turning to food, soda or alcohol in an effort to push the emotions away. Another way may become physical pain or illness when the emotions neurologically affect the chemistry of your body. Or you may find yourself expressing your feelings in ways you don't intend.

Kelley found she lost her temper with her kids for no reason and simmered in anger as she did all the housework after a long day at the office. She did everything for her family, and they didn't seem to appreciate how hard she worked and how much she had sacrificed. When she came to me, she was at the breaking point and felt she had to find a way to take care of herself. She was overweight, bordering on obesity, had high cholesterol and was pre-diabetic. She was sick of doing everything, but she didn't know how to do anything less. How, she asked me, could she change her situation before she grew to hate her husband and her children? She admitted she already hated herself. Since I'm not a psychologist, I didn't attempt to address her marital issues or what in her past led to how she felt. Instead, we focused on her current behaviors, what got in the way of believing she was entitled to make time for her well-being, and ways she could make positive changes that supported her needs.

What she began to discover as she looked at why she didn't choose to put herself first were her false beliefs that she came last in the family, had to carry the responsibility as a breadwinner and needed to be the perfect wife and ideal mother she never had. These beliefs were stretching her too thin and making it impossible to have a life she enjoyed, which made her angry and resentful. These were the feelings she couldn't admit to herself, yet her family was well aware that she wasn't happy and felt somehow responsible for her unhappiness and at a loss for how to improve things. The change needed to start within her.

She decided that she would ask her family to give her fifteen minutes each night to go in her bedroom and close the door for some quiet time. She used this time to do some journaling to process the day and express her feelings. She also made an appointment for a massage. Immediately she felt calmer. She was getting some space to breathe and get in touch with her needs. She started to journal about perfectionism and realized it wasn't what it was cracked up to be and that it didn't really matter as much as she imagined. In our sessions we discussed whether good was good enough, and she began to see that in many areas, it wasn't necessary to aim for perfection and that yes, good was good enough much of the time.

As Kelley began to do more for herself, her family seemed happier and calmer, mirroring the changes in her. They encouraged her to keep doing whatever she needed to feel better, and her husband offered to take care of the housework in the evening so she could attend some yoga and exercise classes. She began losing weight and was able to stop taking her medications, and to her amazement, the love and laughter returned to her marriage and family life. She learned that she had been repressing feelings that were tied to beliefs that didn't support what she really wanted in her life. She also learned that she didn't have to do everything and that her family was happy to help if she let them.

The more you know what you are feeling and allow yourself to express those emotions, the less your feelings run your behaviors, and the better you feel. This can seem frightening because the more you hold on to emotions, the more overwhelming they may seem, and the more you validate them with additional experiences. The natural inclination is to avoid emotions altogether, and, unfortunately, this is encouraged. We are taught to keep our feelings to ourselves, focus on the task at hand and suck it up. And after years of this conditioning, you may have sucked up so much emotion you might be afraid you will explode if you bring any of them up.

Many diabetics I have worked with are in this situation. They get so overwhelmed by feelings about the disease, their bodies and themselves that they shut down and go into denial. What they are facing is scary, and their struggle to manage the disease is often debilitating. On the one hand, diabetics know they have to change their lifestyles to manage their disease, while on the other, they find it incredibly difficult to comply with the list of lifestyle changes they are supposed to do. And when they can't seem to keep up with these changes, they feel guilty, incapable and bad about themselves. After repeating this experience and feeling like a failure or something is terribly wrong with them, it gets harder to get back on track.

Often, it becomes easier to eat comfort foods, skip medications, reduce the frequency of monitoring glucose levels, and pretend the disease doesn't matter. Yet making these choices creates feelings of guilt and a sense of shame, which get repressed. And the more they repress, the less they feel, and the more their health doesn't seem to matter to them. It is not uncommon for diabetics in this state of mind to avoid seeing their doctors. They don't want to get a lecture about the consequences of their actions. They don't want to feel ashamed and belittled for their behavior. Of course they know the ramifications of their choices. They know what the doctor will tell them. They know they have to do better. And that only makes them feel worse and leads to emotional eating and depression. It is no wonder a high percentage of diabetics repress their feelings and pretend everything is fine to the point of going numb. They just don't want to think about the disease. Because diabetes is a silent destroyer with minimal symptoms for the first few years, they can pretend it doesn't really exist.

One of my diabetic clients was so ambivalent that whenever I reminder her that she had diabetes, she would say, "Oh, that's right. I forgot that. It always surprises me when you remind me of that because I don't think of myself as diabetic." Her condition wasn't real for her, even though she also had all the symptoms of syndrome X, which is even more serious than just having diabetes and occurs when you have high blood pressure, high cholesterol, high triglycerides and high blood sugars. She chose not to let the disease register in her mind. She just couldn't take the diagnosis seriously.

Contributing to her mindset was her low self-esteem and a belief that even if she did take care of herself, she would die anyway. The more we discussed her denial of diabetes, the more she looked at these beliefs and got clear on why it did matter to her to have a higher quality life and to be alive for her daughter. She still struggles with her denial, but she has the tools now to identify her feelings and beliefs, and acknowledge the disease so she can make healthier choices.

Another client, Julian, also struggled with denial. He laughed about it, yet he was actually terrified. He had not been able to get his blood sugar levels under control for years, and while he went through periods when he precisely followed all the protocols, he also went through times when he hardly monitored his glucose and binged on junk food. At both times, he felt at a loss because nothing seemed to work, and he felt guilty for not being the model patient, the good eater or the man who could still tackle and get the girls as he did as the football hero back in college.

What doesn't help someone in denial is to remind them that they will pay a consequence for what they are doing. They know diabetes is a terrible way to die and they are on the fast track to death. But to remind them of this not only angers them, it is also the best way to push them further into denial.

Instead, these people need a way to get in touch with what they feel gently and safely without any judgment or fear of repercussions. It is scary to face feelings that carry a lot of pain and anxiety, yet keeping them buried actually makes them appear more frightening than they really are.

An easy way to start to address these feelings, whether you are diabetic, someone dealing with emotional eating or one with feelings that get in the way of making healthier choices, is to acknowledge that your feelings exist. Bring your emotions out into the light and validate what you are really dealing with inside. Acknowledgment helps you start expressing what you are feeling subconsciously so you can start to release those feelings. This step, while initially frightening, can actually give you relief and stop the repression that is keeping you stuck. As one my clients pointed out after a good cry, the actual experience of feeling is not as bad as you think it will be. Yes, you may cry and sob, feel your chest and jaw tighten, clench your fists or even feel a bit sick to your stomach, yet you will also notice you feel better after the emotions get released. You may even feel a sense of relief and completeness. You are opening the door to reclaiming yourself and taking back control of those repressed feelings that have subconsciously driven your behaviors.

The exercise for acknowledging feelings and the source of those feelings that I find most effective and gentle is one I adapted from Linda Spangle's book, *Life is Hard, Food is Easy*, which provides simple and straightforward steps for dealing with emotional eating.

The exercise is this:

When you find yourself overeating, eating when you aren't hungry, avoiding being aerobically active, not taking your medication or vitamins or neglecting yourself, or when you are feeling back pain, a headache or you are dealing with an illness that lingers too long, ask yourself the following:

I am feeling _____ because _____

and what else ...
I am feeling _____ because _____

and what else ...
I am feeling _____ because _____

and what else ...
I am feeling _____ because _____

and what else ...
I am feeling _____ because _____

Don't stop with the first feeling that comes to mind unless you are sure there isn't more to that feeling. In most cases the feeling closest to the surface is a superficial cause of your emotional eating or other behavior. The dominant feeling in play, triggered by the current event, is often more deeply repressed. If you don't get to the bottom of what you feel, you may continue your behaviors in an effort to avoid those deeper feelings. Dig down four or five layers to see what other feelings are buried that is adding fuel to the feeling you first identified.

One of my clients, Christina, was bingeing on sugary foods at work, and she didn't understand why she kept doing that. Here's what she learned when she did this exercise:

I am feeling frightened about losing my job because I know others can do it better.

I am feeling anxious about what my boss thinks because he doesn't acknowledge my work.

I am feeling concerned because I may not be adequate.

I am feeling inadequate because I need approval.

I am feeling I am never good enough because I could never please my father.

Christina was amazed that her overeating had anything to do with her upbringing, yet it made total sense when she saw it in black-and-white. She realized that her father's expectations were one thing, and her ability to do her job was another. She learned that her job was not in danger just because her boss did things that reminded her of her father. This insight helped her be clearer about what was causing her feelings and that she needed to address some old issues with her dad.

By identifying the cause of a feeling and why you are having it, you are also getting at what your needs are. You may need to deal with someone, have a conversation, address an incomplete issue, do something for yourself or change your situation. You may need to do several things, and by looking at all the issues you are dealing with, you get insights into how you can help yourself without turning to food or taking your problems out on yourself.

This approach helps you to identify and release your feelings, understand what created them (which are very often your beliefs) and then figure out what you need to do for yourself. The objective isn't to bring up your feelings so you can go back into your past and try to work them out, as you would in therapy. The objective is to identify the feeling instead of reaching for a distraction such as food or drink. However, if you find you have a need or desire to revisit your past or find that feeling your emotions creates anxiety or other concerns, please consider seeing a professional psychotherapist for assistance.

Identifying Your Beliefs

Beliefs aren't all that easy to identify. Some may be obvious, but many are so ingrained we can't notice them. You may have gone through years of therapy or had considerable healing work and believe you have eradicated your negative beliefs, but they may still linger or be so buried that they are hard to get at. Most of us carry deeply held subconscious beliefs created during the early years of our lives.

I am a good example of this. I started going to therapy when I was eighteen to address issues that started in my childhood, and I continued seeing a therapist until my early forties. In my sessions, I went back and faced many of my feelings, broke free of my shame and got comfortable with myself. Yet it was my last therapist that opened my eyes to my beliefs, which were keeping me stuck. He asked me to do a homework assignment and come back with what I thought was true about my life, myself and my choices. He wanted me to write down my beliefs. As I did this, I found myself surprised by what I was writing. I had so many beliefs that were limiting me, and I could see that my lifestyle and choices were based on them. This was such an eye-opener, and I began to replace those beliefs with new ones that were more positive and aligned with what I wanted in my life. Over the years, I have learned to look into any disappointing or negative experience to further uncover limiting beliefs that have silently made my decisions and created my reality.

A way to zero in on your beliefs is to listen to what you are saying to yourself. Your thoughts are a window into your subconscious, where your beliefs are in charge.

If you spent a day listening to what you said to yourself, you would be shocked by what your inner voice chatters on about, particular when you do things that raise your belief system's critical eye. When I started listening to myself, I discovered I exaggerated and was down right cruel. When I spilled a little bit of coffee while driving, I heard, "Look what you've done! You spilled coffee all over the place." But that wasn't true at all. I didn't spill very much, and it was no big deal. In really hearing what I was saying, I recognized that I was repeating the tone and severity of what was said to me as a child.

As I continued to listen during the next few weeks, I also heard myself say, "How could you be so stupid?"; "I will never be good enough at this"; "Why would anyone want me around?"; "What is wrong with me?"; "I can't do this, so what's the use"; and "You idiot." I couldn't believe I was saying things I knew weren't true, much less things that hurt me so badly. I wouldn't ever say such things to anyone else, no matter how upset they made me. Yet by criticizing myself with harsh judgments over and over again, these criticisms were being locked in as my truth and my story. These distorted views impacted how I felt about myself, how I resisted trying new things, and how close I would let people get to me.

Once I really paid attention to what I was saying internally, I could stop myself midsentence and confront the criticism. I began saying, "Wait a minute, that isn't true," and I then replaced those words with more compassionate and loving ones. It wasn't long before I realized I was seldom criticizing myself, and I was starting to say, "No big deal; everyone has a bad day. Not a problem; that's okay." When I said that, I felt much lighter about what had happened.

Find out what you are saying to yourself by really paying attention when something seems to go wrong or when you do something that isn't perfect. The more you begin to notice and hear your negative self-talk, the more highly tuned you will be any time you criticize yourself. Be prepared to hear the worst. You may even discover you say nasty things about yourself to others who wish you wouldn't be so hard on yourself. People always used to say to me, "Don't be so hard on yourself" or "You don't really mean that." When people say words like this to you, recognize these are indicators that your self-talk is so ingrained you don't even keep it to yourself. Sadly, when you share your self-criticism with others, it can put you further into denial. You might laugh and say, "Yes, I do mean it," without realizing how damaging this response really is. In truth, it separates you from the part of you stung by the remark.

You can often see your negative self-image or critical comments more easily when another person denigrates him or herself. In one of my workshops, a participant referred to himself as a big, fat, disgusting cow, which was painful for the other participants to hear. I asked if he really saw himself that way, and he said no, not really. I encouraged him to listen for the times when he judged himself and to stop when he heard those things — to even say stop if that helped — and check in to the real truth. A week later, he said he was not beating himself up so much and felt more energized. He learned that negative thoughts drain your energy.

Thoughts also validate our beliefs, which represents your understanding and perspective of what you think is true about yourself and the world around you. They provide the basis for how you determine right from wrong and how things should be done. Beliefs are formed by what you are surrounded by and the messages you hear repeatedly as you grow up and go out into the world. They come primarily from your parents and secondarily from your teachers, friends, local customs and the media. Some beliefs are formed to help you survive painful experiences or from your interpretation of how you were treated. Even though you didn't choose which ones to absorb or don't realize you created them to protect yourself, you subconsciously hold them as sacred. These beliefs then become the underlying determinant of what you think and do, even if you once rebelled against them.

Some of the beliefs I took on to protect myself as a child were sabotaging my ability to succeed as an adult, and they stemmed from being surrounded by family members, neighbors and classmates who harshly judged or made fun of me. I came to believe it was not safe to be seen or heard, so I focused on protecting myself from being hurt again and kept people from getting close. Eventually, I understood that it was my beliefs that were hurting me, not the individuals who were judging me.

Fortunately, you can choose which beliefs serve you and which ones you wish to rewrite to support you, once you know what they are. You get to make the rules now.

You can choose to believe you are unlovable, or you can choose to believe you are lovable and find evidence this new belief is true. You can believe only thin women are beautiful, or you can believe women of any size can be just as lovely. You can believe your favorite foods are bad and therefore you are guilty and bad whenever you eat them, or you can believe it is fine to have your favorite food in moderation.

There are so many things you've been told about food, fitness, your body and what you should do to be healthier, and much of is probably not right or, more importantly, not right for you. For example, you have been told through the media that carbohydrates are bad, boot camps are good and you can't be thin enough. Your mother may have instilled in you the practices of dieting and stepping on the scale everyday. Your friends may have encouraged you to diet because this is what they were doing, and your doctor probably backs this practice up. Those in the know have convinced you that exercising for less than thirty or even forty-five minutes isn't worth your time and that to really get in shape you need to go to the gym. And people, at various times in your life, have led you to believe you are unworthy because you are too fat. Am I far off?

Whatever you have come to believe about yourself and what it takes to be healthy, fit and less heavy needs a second look. First, these beliefs need to be brought out into the open, put in perspective and then kept, changed or discarded.

There are several ways to get in touch with your beliefs. You could spend an hour or so and jot down everything you believe to be true about eating, fitness, health and your body. Another approach is to become aware of your self-talk and see how those thoughts are validating your beliefs. A third way is to investigate your feelings and see what beliefs might be behind them.

And last, but not least, is to use the "*I am feeling … because …*" exercise from page 52.

You may find that you don't seem to feel anything specifically or you don't think your problem is caused by a feeling, so you can also ask yourself what you are *thinking* instead of feeling and see where that takes you.

I am thinking _____ because _____

and

That belief comes from

_____

and what else …

I am thinking _____ because _____

and

That belief comes from

_____

and what else …

I am feeling _____ because _____

(You may also bring up associated feelings)

and what else …

In this form of the exercise you are getting at your thoughts, their underlying beliefs and where those beliefs were established. Knowing the source of your beliefs can be helpful in understanding why you hold onto then and giving yourself permission to release and replace them.

As you become aware of your beliefs, you can look back to see where they came from to put them in perspective. At some point in your life, they may have served you well. The question now is, do they still serve you, or are they holding you back from living a full and better life?

Tiffany always wanted to eat something the minute she got done working. She started thinking, as she got in the elevator after work, about what she wanted to eat. On her drive home, she would stop and get her favorite cheese sticks, ice cream sandwiches, donuts or whatever she thought looked good. She would start eating her goodies in the car, and once she was home, she would feel compelled to finish them off so she wouldn't have them in the house.

She admitted she didn't stop for food because she was hungry. Instead, she realized, she thought she deserved a reward because she had worked hard during the day. She grew up, as so many of us did, getting food as a reward after school, for doing homework or for getting something else done. She realized she didn't need to get rewarded this way. She could find other ways to reward herself. She also realized this was a habit and she associated food with ending her work day, which helped her to change her thinking and her behavior.

What was tougher for her was dealing with food after a dinner party. She's Italian and loves to cook and entertain. Yet after her guests left one of her parties, she would find herself eating whatever food was leftover, no matter how much remained. She was compelled to do it, and she didn't really know why. As we talked through it and did the "*I am feeling or I am thinking … because …*" exercise, she said that she couldn't throw food away and couldn't save leftovers, so she really had no other choice. These were beliefs she got from her mother, who drilled it into her head that throwing food out was wasteful and that leftovers created a bad smell in the refrigerator and in the house. This created a no-win situation whenever she cooked. I helped her see that she could now set new rules for her house and choose new beliefs that suited her needs and values. She began to experiment with throwing food out and found a way to justify it by looking at the real costs of eating extra food. These costs included her sugar depressions, the expense of medication for depression and treating pre-diabetes, lost productivity when she was too sick to work the following day and, in the long-term, becoming less healthy.

Creating new beliefs is easier than you might think. We hold our beliefs in our subconscious, which holds onto whatever you tell it to with conviction and repetition. The subconscious is much like a database that has no interest in what data is stored in it. You can replace an old belief with a new one by writing over the file. But you have to rewrite it enough to fully replace the old version. Another analogy that I once heard is the subconscious is like an LP record that has a deep groove where a needle has played over and over. To replace such a deep groove, you have to create another one just as deep by playing the new belief over and over until the needle stays in it and doesn't skip back to the old groove.

When you create a new belief, you need to repeat it and be conscious of it frequently enough that you come to really own it as your truth. Sometimes all it takes is proof that it works for you, and you can eradicate the old fact with a new one overnight. More often, the new belief requires repeating regularly. This repetition is called affirming a new truth. Tiffany created a new belief that throwing out food saved her money. This became her new affirmation.

Affirmations are very helpful in changing beliefs because they reinforce and affirm what you are now choosing to believe as true. They are positive statements that validate what you know is best for you or what you want for yourself, and you read or say them repeatedly over a period of days or weeks until they really sink in and creates that deeper groove. Your affirmations might be "I am enough"; "I am successful"; "It is best to throw out food I don't need"; or "I can eat my favorite foods whenever I want them in moderation because I can always get more." Note that you can always change these affirmations and improve upon them as you make changes or as you discover what works even better. You may not fully believe these new affirmations initially, but the more you repeat them, the more you reprogram your belief system and the more they will become your new perspective and reality.

Reaching Inner Wisdom

In addition to understanding your thoughts and beliefs (your mental self) and your feelings (your emotional self), you can learn much more about yourself by tuning into your body (your physical self) and listening to your heart and intuition (your spiritual self). Each part of the self is connected with the others, and as you change patterns in one area, you affect the others directly — either positively or negatively.

Our physical, mental, emotional and spiritual selves offer pathways to our inner wisdom. This wisdom can guide, inspire and motivate you to make positive changes for yourself and help you gain greater clarity about what is important. Many of us have lost our connection to what really matters and what we value. Instead, we focus on all the obligations we take on and what has to be done. We get caught up in our schedule of to-dos and lose sight of our purpose, passion and preferences.

When we live out of integrity with our values, we don't listen to our hearts. We also shut down mentally, emotionally, physically and spiritually. I know this firsthand because I am a former workaholic and a daughter trying to please my father. I made choices that were about pleasing others and trying to be what I thought others would respect and value. I was completely disconnected from my feelings, beliefs, body and soul for most of my life. I was convinced I couldn't rely on my own inner wisdom because I didn't think I had any.

Yet we all have wisdom. For each of us, the journey to fully connect with our bodies and our true selves takes different paths and evolves at a different pace. For some it starts with physical awareness, which opens the door for greater insight. For others it starts with a spiritual or emotional opening. Fortunately, any connection with yourself gives you more access to your inner wisdom and helps you make choices that are more aligned with your needs and wants.

Tuning in to Your Body

Your body sends you lots of signals in the form of pain, discomfort, hunger, fullness, low energy and weight gain. Many of us disregard these signals and deny they exist. When you do this, you set yourself up to feel even worse, and you put your body at risk for injury, illness and disease. These signals are a reminder to take care of yourself. Additional signals come from medical tests that indicate when hormones are out of balance, cholesterol or blood pressure is too high or blood sugar levels are in the danger zone.

Your body also lets you know that you are out of balance when it is overweight or when body fat and muscle are out of proportion. If your lean body mass is low because you have a high percentage of fat, your metabolism will slow down and you won't feel energized. When you lose your muscle, you won't be able to lift as much, you won't look toned and you will have less shock absorption in your knees and joints. When your hormones are out of balance, you will notice that you don't feel as well as when they are in balance.

Georgette was finding she didn't feel well for two weeks of each month and thought the feeling might be tied to premenstrual syndrome because she craved more sugar and salt. Yet she also noticed that if she didn't eat every few hours, she would feel faint, and being active always made her feel better. She had been tested for diabetes regularly, but she was always told that she was fine and just had hypoglycemia (a condition in which blood sugar levels dip very low). As we talked about her observations in one of our sessions, I suggested she monitor her blood glucose to see if her low levels were in response to extremely high blood sugar readings after she ate. Bingo. She discovered that was exactly what was going on. She had reactive hypoglycemia. So she began eating more balanced meals to regulate her blood sugars, and immediately she experienced a difference in how she felt.

Pain is another signal you need to pay close attention to, particularly if its cause has gone undiagnosed. Many people walk around for months or even years with pain from overusing a muscle, having postural imbalances or living with an injury. They just live with the pain and ultimately become more inactive and both emotionally and physically debilitated. I did the same thing a number of years ago. I tore a tendon while exercising after disregarding the aches that gave me an initial warning, and the physical therapist I went to see said I had been an injury waiting to happen. If you disregard or accept pain, you too may be susceptible to injury.

Lucinda could barely get up or down a flight of stairs and walked as if she were crippled. She'd been getting worse for years, and it frightened her. She wasn't old enough to be so out of shape, and she blamed herself for letting her condition go on for so long. As a result of her feelings, she wouldn't go to the doctor. She was too embarrassed and afraid of what she would learn. Instead she became increasingly housebound and dependent on her husband and children, which was the last thing she wanted. Her pride and fear were so strong that she subconsciously chose a restricted and poor quality of life over getting the help she needed. With a better understanding of what was driving her behavior, she did see her doctor, who prescribed physical therapy exercises to minimize the pain and get her moving again.

Feeling full or ravenously hungry are also important signals. There is no better appetite suppressant than feeling full, but if you don't stop to notice when you get full, you will end up overeating. For some people, this is a nightly occurrence. On the flip side, it is equally common to ignore hunger signals. You may choose not to eat when you get hungry because you believe not eating is a way to lose weight, you are too busy to stop or that food isn't readily available when you feel hungry. Ignoring either signal (fullness or hunger) slows down metabolism, leads to weight gain, negatively impacts blood sugar levels and creates carbohydrate cravings and bingeing.

Stress has its own signals. Being stressed because you are trying to do too much or you are not taking care of yourself, can lead to anxiety, insomnia, chronic pain, headaches, illness or other maladies. Stress can also lead you to feel helpless, out of control or over reactive. The symptoms of stress are red flags telling you that you aren't taking care of your physical or emotional needs.

For years I lived with my chronic fatigue, irritable bowel syndrome, daily nausea, severe back pain and then significant weight gain. I knew I worked too much and was unhappy in a relationship, but I didn't understand that my physical symptoms were tied to my choices. My reaction to these signals was to just keep putting one foot in front of the other and do what I felt I had to do each day. I didn't look at my symptoms as anything but physical problems that I was helpless to do anything about. I couldn't have been more wrong. They had everything to do with the way I was running my life and my unwillingness to see how my choices played a role in my health.

Instead I turned to doctors, but they couldn't help me. I even went to see a renowned specialist in Philadelphia for a series of gastrointestinal tests that lasted several days to get a better opinion about why I was chronically nauseated. The physician found nothing abnormal and wondered whether I was under considerable stress. I said no, not really, and left the building frustrated. I was truly blind to what was happening in my life. It took multiple rounds of being bedridden for months at a time before I started to see that I was pushing myself too hard and not taking care of myself. I hadn't been very active, taken a vacation or worked less than ten-to-twelve hours a day in years. The problem was that being under enormous stress was normal to me, so I couldn't see it. Not until I changed my lifestyle and made my health a priority did my symptoms completely disappear.

Margot wasn't so lucky, as she shared once with the listeners on my radio show. She was a type A go-getter who didn't let anything stop her from doing what she had to do in her career. Even waking up one morning and finding that she couldn't see out of one eye did not stop her from going to her appointments. Nor did she stop when she noticed weakness in her legs. She didn't stop until her body made it very clear she didn't have a choice but to stop, and she was diagnosed with multiple sclerosis. She finally got the message loud and clear, and to this day, she believes that her illness is a result of living a life of chronic stress. Many others who have debilitating illnesses have wondered the same thing. This hasn't been proven, yet it is likely that these people suppressed their immune systems' abilities to ward off the onset of their diseases.

You don't have to wind up in the hospital, receive a diagnosis of disease, get sick or get derailed by an injury to start paying attention. Get to know what your body is wisely trying to tell you and then determine the best course of action. It doesn't matter if someone else thinks you should push yourself to an extreme measure if you know, or even suspect, that action isn't right for you.

Listening to Your Heart

When you take the time to reflect on what really matters to you, instead of what you are supposed to do or how you need to earn a living, you get reconnected to your values and your heart. When most people do this, they find what they value is: being happy, fulfilling their purpose, giving back to society, helping others, enjoying themselves, feeling content, being healthy and fit to do anything they want, and having freedom to make their own choices.

Similarly, when people are surveyed about their dreams, the most common dreams are fulfilling a purpose and being slim, fit or healthy. These dreams go hand in hand; you can't easily live out your dream for fulfillment if you don't have your health or you aren't fit enough to pursue your purpose. Additionally, without your dreams, you may lose your desire to live and your spiritual, mental, emotional and physical health. You won't care to take good care of yourself, if you don't have hopes and dreams.

Feeling good about oneself and having an ability to contribute to others, is something most people long for, even when these desires are repressed. As you get older, your inner dreams come into your consciousness and help you see the contrast between how you are currently living and what your heart and soul desire. For some people, it takes a midlife crisis, medical trauma or serious illness to see what matters. For others, who never acknowledge their dreams, they will often further repress their needs. They may give up and succumb to depression, self-pity and disease.

My midlife crisis occurred the last time I was bedridden. I was getting burned out on my career, to which I had given most of my life. I was terrified I no longer felt the passion for my high tech career, as a highly respected industry analyst. I had loved the industry and my role in it, and it had been my identity for more than twenty years. I couldn't imagine doing anything else, yet part of me no longer cared about being an analyst. I had burned the candle at both ends for too long, and I was physically a wreck. I was also gaining a significant amount of weight and was unable to control the weight gain with dieting, which also terrified me. It was one of the darkest and scariest times of my life, and it took a yearlong sabbatical of self-care to understand what interested and mattered to me. I spent that year exercising regularly, gardening, cooking healthy meals and doing some volunteer projects. These became new passions for me, and these activities helped me get in touch with what I really cared about, which was my health and a healthy lifestyle.

For those like me, who have survived great suffering and been awakened to their own truth, they too have pulled themselves out of their darkness with a determination to live and thrive. These people don't take things for granted, and they don't give up. They tend to value everything they have, even if their physical bodies have been compromised. There are countless stories of people who have been in wheelchairs, given little time to live or been told they will never function again, who have found inner strength, perseverance and healing practices to bring their bodies back into a state of health no one would have expected. These people focus on having the best lives they can, taking better care of themselves and feeling grateful for their lessons.

Margot says she is grateful now that she has multiple sclerosis because she discovered the importance of living a balanced lifestyle and taking good care of herself. She has also done what most would say is impossible. She has slowly and steadily regained her strength and no longer spends her days in a wheelchair. She can now walk again, swim and go to Curves. She got strong by connecting to her spiritual center, visualizing herself moving, asking for help, believing in herself and experimenting with different types of movement programs.

Maureen Whitehouse, author of *Soul-Full Eating*, and Marian Baker, who wrote *Wake Up Inspired*, were also guests on my show. They shared their own stories of how they overcame being out of balance and then connected with their inner wisdom. Maureen was a former international model, who starved herself to compete with other models in an industry that was in conflict with her values. She did some soul searching and began to question what starving and her other forms of dysfunctional eating were doing to her body and to herself. She realized in the process of that soul searching she had lost herself to the profession. That realization provided the shift to regain her authenticity and honor her spirit. She then had greater health and happiness, and she was able to model successfully for many more years.

Marian was at the top of her game as an advertising executive, when she began to feel something was very wrong. She knew the feeling was more than the physical symptoms she was dealing with. She was getting a persistent sensation that something wasn't right, as if her insides were knocking and asking, "can we talk?" She felt restless, out of balance and unfulfilled. This feeling put her on a healing quest, which led her to discover how to open up to what her heart was telling her and follow its guidance. She experienced many insights and a shift in perspective. She discovered that her physical health was inseparable from her spiritual and mental well-being, and that she needed to focus on her self-care and quality of life.

My mentor, Marcia Wieder, followed her heart out of a high-powered position in Washington, D.C. to San Francisco where she pursued her passion for making dreams come true. She wrote *Making Your Dreams Come True, Doing Less and Having More,* and *Dreams are Whispers from the Soul.* She also developed the first certification Dream Coach® program, and she has trained hundreds of coaches, including me, how to guide people in discovering their purpose and be in action to follow their dreams. Her training is now the foundation of her organization Dream University®. She is happier than she could have once imagined, and she is living her life in alignment with her heart.

When you listen to your heart and connect to your spiritually, you often discover you want to live your life more fully, contribute to others through your purpose and follow your dreams. You become more connected with all parts of your being and discover the need for alignment between your physical, mental, emotional and spiritual states. And when that happens, you are guided more easily by your inner wisdom, and you are more inclined toward healthier choices and a healthy way of living.

Choices without Deprivation or a Need for Perfection

Knowing yourself well helps you to make choices that are best for you and gives you the confidence to stand up for your own way of doing things. This self-determination is important in a world of unlimited options, conflicting advice, varying types of experts and a wide array of fitness, health and diet programs.

By choosing things you enjoy most, you have a greater chance of wanting to do them. This is what Nick Yphantides, a physician who nearly lost his life from being unhealthy and severely obese, realized after he was diagnosed with testicular cancer and took a sabbatical across America in pursuit of baseball games and a healthier lifestyle. He focused on being active and making healthier choices during his trip, and he came to understand that being healthy isn't about dieting or exercising. It is about living and having fun. His insights transformed his thinking and choices, and when he got back he was 270 pounds lighter. He wrote *My Big Fat Greek Diet* in order to share his story and help others discover a more enjoyable approach to healthy living than dieting and exercising.

Many people are discovering the same thing. Shann started working out in a gym when she first realized her lifestyle was out of control. Going to the gym helped get her moving, but it didn't hold her interest. She decided what she really wanted was a way to relax, be outdoors and have more fun and variety. She started to do yoga and Pilates, then she added martial arts and months later she included running and snowboarding into her activities. Her goal wasn't to achieve perfection. It was to give herself permission to take care of herself doing what she liked best, and from this permission she discovered how to enjoy being healthy and active.

Discovering Choices

Despite what you've been told, there are no bad foods and there are lots of ways to be aerobic to burn fat. You don't have to use gym equipment or go to the gym for exercise, unless that works for you. You don't have to give up chocolate or your favorite foods, unless they don't agree with you. It is a myth you have to eat a certain way to lose weight or work out using specific types of routines to get back into shape and be fit. If it were true, more people would be successful.

What works is finding foods and activities you like that are healthier than what you are eating and doing now. You don't have to make drastic changes or push yourself to choose things you don't want. That is exactly what doesn't work for most people.

The best way to improve your eating habits, for example, is to focus on what you want to eat and then to make small adjustments in how it is prepared so it is healthier. When clients ask me what they should have for their meals, I turn it around and ask them what they enjoy eating for breakfast, lunch, dinner and various snacks. Then I explain they can find ways to eat those things in a healthier way by reducing the saturated fat and simple carbohydrates. This is easily done by substituting some of the ingredients, finding foods with less of these nutrients, or switching to healthier brands.

When I take clients to the grocery store to learn how to select healthier foods they will enjoy, we often start by finding foods for breakfast. When I met Mandy at the store, I asked her what she liked to eat in the morning and she said, "I love eggs, bacon and toast, but I know I can't have these because of the carbohydrates and fat." I told her the belief she couldn't have these foods may not be true, and I suggested we go look at her bacon options. There were many different types of bacon, from lean turkey bacon to thick slabs of smoked bacon, and I told her to pick out a couple of the leanest options — with the least amount of saturated fat — she would want to try. The goal was to find leaner bacon she liked, and the only way to find out was to buy them and taste them. The bacon she didn't like, I recommended she throw out instead of feeling obligated to eat it.

As we found with the bacon, there were several options for eggs with less saturated fat, from egg substitutes to eggs higher in Omega 3. She could also choose to cook with more egg whites than yolks to reduce the amount of fat. In the bread isle, we found dozens of whole grain breads that were high in complex carbohydrates. We also looked for cereals for higher amounts of complex carbohydrates and lower amounts of sugar, which we found the specialty cereal section. I gave her some rules of thumb to make her cereal selections, which was five or less grams of sugar per serving and at least three grams of fiber and of protein. We put in her cart any cereal that met those criteria and that she might like, and when we were done, she picked just four of them to take home to try. She discovered she liked many of these healthier options, and they tasted just as good as the cereal that was much higher in simple carbohydrates.

The similar approach can be used to choose fitness activities that are enjoyable. If you love to hike, explore the most enjoyable way you can do that within your fitness ability. If you prefer volleyball, pick that activity. If you love to dance, focus on selecting a type you enjoy. Be imaginative and think outside the box. A great resource is the magazine *Experience Life*, which has the most open-minded and delightful perspective on fitness. Each month the magazine has exciting stories about people being active in every way imaginable, including kayaking, soccer, skiing, hiking, martial arts, swimming, running, basketball, dance, tennis and yoga.

Once, when I was working at a booth at a diabetes conference, a woman approached and asked me what she could do in the winter months when it was too cold for walking. She didn't have much money to buy equipment or join classes, so she didn't do any activity during the winter. I asked her what she had enjoyed doing when she was younger, and she said not much. Yet as we kept talking, I learned she had been the hula hoop queen back in junior high. I told her she could get a great aerobic workout with a hula hoop, and it wouldn't cost her more than a few dollars or take up much space at home. She was delighted. She remembered loving her hula hoop, and when I later saw her in the bathroom, she was beaming with excitement. She said she had been thinking about the hula hoop since we talked earlier that day, and she couldn't wait to get started.

Any activity that gets you moving and keeps your heart rate up in the fat-burning zone is a wonderful way to be aerobic. Information about the aerobic fat-burning zone is on page 92. If you want to be active outdoors, there are lots of things you can do. If you prefer being part of a group, there are many types of outdoor classes, walking groups and fitness programs. Instead of thinking about what exercise or a workout is supposed to be, think of what sounds like fun and where you can go to do it.

For people with physical limitations, there are probably more options than you imagine, including ways to be aerobic sitting in a chair. Chair aerobics is basically raising and waving your arms in a rhythmic motion while moving your legs back and forth as you stay seated, and those motions will get your heart rate up into the aerobic zone. I was surprised just how much exertion is involved when I tried it for myself.

Overcoming Deprivation

No doubt, at one time or another, you've been told very specifically what you should and shouldn't eat or do by your parents, doctor, nutritionist, trainer or friends or from magazine articles. Most likely you attempted to do just as you were told, up until you unintentionally deviated from these instructions or felt driven to do the opposite of what you were told. If so, you were reacting in a predictable manner.

When you are told you can't have something, you want it more. When you are forced to do something you don't like to do, you will likely drag your feet or do what's been asked under duress, and then very often you will find a way to quit doing it at all. Most people resent and rebel against being deprived of what they want or for how they want to feel.

When you rebel against a restriction, you will tend to do the opposite of what is being enforced. Think of a diet you've been on and the list of foods that were not allowed. If they were foods you loved, you likely felt a pang for them that developed into a craving or obsession. As soon as you could get your hands on these foods, you probably overindulged as if you couldn't get enough. When you overindulge, it is as if your inner teenager is rebelling against a restrictive parent, and knowing the behavior is really bad, you eat even more. It is common for dieters to overeat when a diet ends and for those on highly restrictive diets to further binge. Some dieters get into a cycle of dieting and bingeing for years, which can wreck havoc on their metabolism and their self-esteem.

Mary, another guest on my show, started restricting her food intake back in high school when she began obsessing about her weight. Her restriction led to days of skipping all meals only to overeat or binge the following days. The fasting and bingeing became a roller coaster of feeling self-righteous on the up days and self-hatred on the down ones. While she restricted herself to gain control over her body, she only got heavier and more depressed. She rode this dieting-deprivation ride for years, unaware that she had an unhealthy relationship with food and was perpetually stuck in a pattern of disordered eating.

Having an unhealthy relationship can also happen with exercise. If you agree to do a fitness program or you purchase a piece of equipment you really don't enjoy, you will likely hate doing it and dread the next time you are supposed to do it. Soon you will be skipping appointments or using the equipment as a place on which to hang things. Exercising or not, you won't feel good about either, and you will be inclined to deny these feelings. Inevitability, just as with a diet, you will probably quit and do nothing. Doing nothing and resisting the idea of working out is a form of deprivation backlash. You are depriving yourself of enjoyment or doing something you prefer, and once you experience the backlash of resistance and ambivalence it may take months or years to be motivated to get active again.

Resistance and ambivalence happens frequently to people who hoped a boot camp would whip them back into shape. I got a call from Lynn after she had enrolled her family in a boot camp program. She was concerned by their behavior when the program ended. She had hired a trainer to come to the house, and the first thing the trainer did was clear out the foods not allowed on the program. Then he created a daily boot camp program that included a severely restricted diet plan and an intense fitness regimen similar to what is done for the TV reality shows.

After a few months, the family began to rebel and Lynn decided the program was expecting too much of her family and stopped it. What happened next she didn't anticipate. Everyone started to binge on junk food and resist doing any type of physical activity. The success they each had doing the boot camp was being replaced with significant weight gain, lower energy and feelings of guilt. The whole experience left a bad taste in their mouths, and Lynn was scared it was going to be impossible to encourage healthier behaviors again.

The moral of the story is instead of being restrictive and depriving yourself of enjoyment, give yourself permission to choose enjoyable healthy options.

Rethinking Perfection

It is nearly impossible to be perfect, yet perfection is what many of us have come to expect of ourselves. We expect that when we've been given a diet or fitness regimen to follow, we are required to fully and perfectly comply with the rules. We are taught repeatedly in our lives to either do something right or face the consequences. Most of us have been berated, asked to account for why we didn't do as was asked, and threatened with a penalty.

What if you were expected to do less and celebrated for small improvements instead? What if you were satisfied to set smaller goals that were realistic enough to always succeed? And what if you were allowed to pick what you wanted to do because only you know yourself best and what you can really achieve?

This freedom of taking baby steps and having personal choice is how Anne, a guest on my show, succeeded to get fit beyond her wildest imagination. Her initial goal was to lose five pounds, and she was happy with that goal. She wanted to fit back into a size 26 pant comfortably, which had become too snug. She surprised herself by losing twenty pounds after three months of walking on the treadmill, so she set another goal for five more pounds. She easily reached that goal and kept setting new goals that were within her reach. She never pushed herself to lose a hundred pounds, yet four years later she had lost a total of ninety-three pounds and realized how far she had come. What kept her going was feeling successful and having choices. She didn't want to be told what to do, and instead, she asked for guidance and then made her own decisions based on what felt right to her. Anne allowed herself to set small goals that were realistic and to make choices that best suited her. Because of that permission, she surpassed her own expectations and discovered a passion for fitness that led to body-building competitions and size 4 outfits.

Giving yourself permission to choose activities you enjoy, the pace you feel comfortable with and goals you can reach, changes the rules of fitness. This fresh perspective is just what many people need to succeed at getting fit and healthy. Instead of expecting yourself to perfectly adhere to someone else's overbearing demands, pick a fitness activity and an amount of time you can do fairly easily and progress to doing more from that point — one small success after another. Soon enough you will be achieving more than you thought possible, and you will have a lot to be proud of.

Confidence and Control are Priceless

Feeling confident and in control is what most of us want, and when you have those feelings you also feel invincible, energized and good about yourself. Self-confidence also changes your attitude. You become more positive and focused on what you can do rather than on what you should do. Clients often tell me they have achieved this confidence while working with me, after having integrated the three Cs into their lifestyle.

Once you have achieved greater confidence and control in your behaviors toward food, exercising and self-care, it becomes easier to trust your own inner wisdom and give yourself what you need. You also stop feeling pressured by other people's rules, shoulds or judgment. You now know best.

Part Three

Creating a Healthier Lifestyle That Feels Good

Being Active and Fit

Eating Healthier with Satisfaction

Creating a Healthier Lifestyle That Feels Good

There is a difference between wanting a healthier lifestyle and creating one you can stick with. You may understand the rationale behind the 3 Cs, but you may not see how you can use them to successfully change your behaviors about food and physical fitness. In this section I am going to walk you through the steps to becoming fit and eating healthier using the 3 Cs, so you can easily create a healthy lifestyle that is enjoyable, motivating and satisfying.

Being Active and Fit

The common belief is you have to exercise to be healthy and fit. You can also be healthy and fit by choosing to be more active. It isn't just a play on words, although their meanings do overlap. Exercise is defined as bodily or mental exertion, whereas being active is defined as being engaged in action or in a state of motion. The difference is a change in mindset and the types of activities you choose. For those that resist the idea of exercising, this difference opens up more options to become fit.

As with the term "workout", as I discussed earlier in the book, "exercise" to most people sounds like work or a chore they would rather put off until tomorrow and often that is just what happens. When people think about *exercising*, they don't just think *working out*. Many will tell you they also associate exercise with the phrases: boring, sweating, have to, hate it, drudgery, working hard, going for the burn, don't do it, not good at it, the gym, or feels great. Those who tend to have negative associations with the word "exercise" likely have had bad experiences, didn't grow up exercising, believe exercise has to be extreme, or can only think of exercise within the confines of a gym, physical education class or fitness program.

When I ask people what comes to mind when I say "being active," they respond more positively. Being active feels good to them, and it is something they want to be able to do for the rest of their lives. They associate being active with outdoor activities, going places, having fun, feeling alive, remaining independent and having an active lifestyle.

Stuart is a good example of someone who responds better to the idea of being active. He was feeling anxious about having to exercise because it felt like an assignment. He had many negative associations about exercise from his childhood. When I asked him how he felt about being active, his tone completely changed. He said he liked to be active and was enthusiastic about being outside walking, hiking and gardening. For him, it was a positive thing that he wanted more of in his life. Whereas exercise was something he didn't feel he was that good at, would have to develop a skill for and frankly was resistant to doing.

Not everyone feels that way. Some people love the idea of exercising and look forward to creating specific gym programs and workout routines. I tend to fall into this camp and still enjoy my StairMaster and strength training time. Others can't wait to sign up for the latest boot camp and love pushing themselves to the limit. Everyone is different, and that is the point. For those who dread exercising, they can choose ways of being active that feel more welcoming and positive.

Whether you prefer exercising or being active, once you embrace either one you will discover the reward of doing something that feels so good you can't imagine not doing it. I am one who finally embraced it, but for the first forty years of my life I couldn't imagine enjoying physical activity because I equated it with exercise and had hated the times in my past when I attempted it. I tried to get out of exercise obligations in my teens, dabbled in exercise programs during my twenties, successfully avoided exercise for most of my thirties and discovered a passion for it at forty-five, three years after I had created an enjoyable way to add exercise into my lifestyle.

What I discovered at forty-four, the second year I stuck with exercising, was the benefits of feeling energized, strong, toned and generally calm and positive, as well as how good being active felt and how much I missed those benefits if I didn't do it. Exercising regularly changed my life and became my priority. I built my day around being active and exercising, instead of trying to fit it into my schedule. Making exercise the priority is just what other people tell me they do when they discover how much they value having it in their life.

The way to successfully and easily incorporate exercise into your life is by first choosing activities and a pace you can comfortably do without pushing yourself too much. After you've been successful doing those activities at that pace for a while, you will discover you have a desire to see if you can push yourself to do a bit more or to try other types of physical activities. Once you get excited by your new abilities and activities, and how good it feels, you will also discover a greater desire to include fitness in your daily lifestyle.

For some people, the mindset shift from resisting activity to loving it, or even from being okay with exercising to fully embracing it, can happen in a few months. For others, the change in mindset can take much longer. The initial shift starts by taking action. As you have probably experienced, this initial enthusiasm can end as quickly as it starts. Very often motivation is lost at the first disruption that keeps you from reaching your goals, or it is lost in the prospect of having to reach for those goals again after the momentum has been broken. For many people, months or even years can go by after a disruption occurs, before they can generate enough interest to try being active again. I have good news for these people. There is a more motivating approach of becoming active, whether you want to call it exercising or being active, that doesn't take so much effort to start or maintain. The approach is based on the 3 Cs.

Applying the 3 Cs to Fitness

If you have ever exercised regularly, even if for a short period of time, take a moment and reflect on that experience. If you are like most people, you will probably recall how focused you were on doing what you were asked to do and how hard you tried to do everything asked of you correctly, even if the exercise hurt or pushed you too hard. You may have believed that experiencing some pain or discomfort was good because it meant something good was happening in your body and you were getting results. Or you may have deliberately looked for a trainer or instructor that would push you really hard, so you could feel you had a good workout. Yet nine times out of ten, feeling pushed or pushing yourself to the point of pain and exhaustion will lead to injury, feeling overwhelmed and resistance. Many of my clients have had experiences with one of these outcomes in their past, which has kept them from pursuing regular activity again.

Consciousness without Judgment

When you rely on others to tell you what you should do, or if you carry beliefs about what a worthwhile fitness program requires (such as a minimum of forty-five minutes of cardio fitness at a pace where you can barely talk), you are less likely to tune into the signals your body is sending you. Instead you will tune out your own instincts and focus more on the judgmental self-talk that will try to force you to comply with what deep down you know isn't right for you.

Years ago I had a personal trainer who thought it was his job to make me do what I didn't believe was possible. There is a fine line between helping people achieve what they don't think they can do and pushing them too hard to reach a goal. I didn't know the difference. When I questioned him or told him I didn't think I could do something because of my back, he told me not to be a baby and just do it. So I did. I wanted to please him and be good. I wanted him to tell me I'd done a good job. Yet I paid a price for acquiescing. I had severe back problems and spent as much money seeing my chiropractor as I did my trainer. And I wasn't the only one. My chiropractor's business was thriving on account of my trainer and others like him. What is sad to me now is that I knew there were certain things that aggravated my back, but I let the trainer bully me around thinking I couldn't say no.

Only you know what your body is experiencing, and you do have the right to say no to anyone who is pushing you too hard or to the point of pain. Fortunately many trainers and instructors do know the difference, but not all of them.

Being aware of how you feel physically takes practice both while you are being active or exercising and when you are going about your day. The awareness starts with being conscious of your breathing and your energy levels as well as any soreness, cramps, sharp pains, stiffness or strange feelings. Notice without judgment what feels good and what doesn't. You may find that breathlessness, hyperventilating, gripping the bars of a cardiovascular exercise machine or straining to keep up a pace doesn't feel good, and that is worthwhile to notice.

If it doesn't feel good, it isn't doing you much good either. The belief of no-pain-no-gain has been proven false and damaging. Instead, you will be more successful in improving your fitness level by limiting your exertion to a more moderate pace and challenging your body periodically with higher intensities that don't hurt or strain you. In time you will know when and how to push yourself a bit more. It is just as important to your fitness success to also slow down or take a day off when your body needs the rest.

When Madeline decided to go back to the gym, she realized her hips got sore easily. She discovered quickly that using the elliptical training equipment along with some stretching reduced the pain. She also noticed she could comfortably only do about fifteen minutes on the elliptical machine, so she decided to use the other fifteen minutes she had walking the treadmill. Soon she felt much better and wanted to do more on the machines, so she began to increase the intensity on the equipment and her time, while paying attention to how her body felt. Weeks later when she got sick, she gave herself permission to take the time she needed to rest. When she went back to the gym afterward, she didn't push herself the first couple of days to do more than an easy pace on both pieces of equipment. The following week she felt great, and was right back in the swing of things and ready to add back in the time and intensity to her routine.

After Gabriella suffered severe sciatica and back pain for four months, which kept her from going to the gym and made it difficult to walk, she eased back into her routine by letting her back decide how much it wanted to do. She told me, "I would look at a piece of [strengthening] equipment and ask my back what it thought was best before deciding to use it." I was so proud of her for this. She was really listening to what was right for her body and not apologizing to herself or anyone else about her limits. In some instances she got a clear, "Not doing that." and in others she was intuitively guided to use the lowest settings or no weight resistance at all. Afterward she felt fine, and she felt confident about easily rebuilding her gym routine and physical strength.

Paying attention to your body is also important to notice if you feel any discomfort on the days in between exercising or being active, particularly when you first start up again. Lots of people get sidelined by injuries when they resume being active because they do too much too soon, and you often don't know you've gotten sore or hurt until the next day or until it catches up with you. My client Karl thought he could walk forty-five minutes four or more times a week, but five weeks into this routine his knees began bothering him and soon he couldn't walk at all. I had cautioned him about overdoing it, but he had felt fine at the time.

By the time I started coaching Demi, I knew of enough people who experienced physical problems from doing too much too soon, that I was telling clients to set less ambitious goals when they started their routines and to progress more carefully. I warned them not to do more than their bodies were prepared to handle. Demi took this to heart, yet she got so enthusiastic about her walks that she doubled the amount of time planned because she felt so good as she walked she didn't want to stop. Her long walks seemed fine for the first few months, but then we began noticing she was getting sick frequently. What we realized was she was walking too much, so she planned to cut back. But she didn't get the chance to see how well that would work. The following week she got very sick and soon after she had a fall that derailed her efforts for a long period of time — and sadly for so long she lost her motivation for getting started again. She finally got motivated a year later.

There is nothing worse than being ready to take action, getting started, finding a good routine and rhythm and seeing some results, only to be disrupted by an injury or illness that throws you completely off course. Disruptions are a motivation killer that will knock the wind out of your sails. It is better to start a new activity off slowly and easily, and then to progress at a moderate pace while paying attention to what your body is wisely trying to tell you.

Clarity through Understanding

The more you know about yourself, your body and how various types of activities help you get healthier, fitter and stronger, the easier it is to make better decisions for yourself. What you don't know can hurt you or reduce the chance you will be successful.

Clarity — the second C — starts off by listening to your body and understanding what you need. If you overdo an activity and find you are sore or hurting, the best course of action is give yourself a chance to recover. Recovery means taking enough time off so you don't have any pain (muscle soreness from strength training being the exception), and if you are in pain to ice, elevate the injured part of your body, and perhaps add an anti-inflammatory cream or pill. Don't try to be too active too soon, or you may find your injury is worsened. Allow yourself the time you need to heal, and then when you start back to your routine start off easy. It is fine, and often ideal, to reduce the amount of time and intensity the first few weeks. If all goes well, you can kick your routine back up to where you were before you took a break. Soon you will be back into the swing of your routine and will hardly remember that you took some time out, just as Madeline learned.

Be aware that muscle soreness from strengthening is normal within twenty-four to forty-eight hours of doing resistance conditioning, and the soreness can last a couple of days. This is common when you first add strengthening to your routine and seldom happens once you are doing it regularly.

If you have ongoing pain, then see your doctor or a physical therapist to determine the best course of treatment. If you wait too long, the problem could be tougher to address and take longer to heal. Very often the pain is the result of muscle imbalances, which means certain muscles are tight and others are loose and weak. This happens when you use the same group of muscles repeatedly as you go about our daily life to the exclusion of using other ones, such as your back and abdominal muscles. When your muscles are stronger on one side of a joint and weaker on the other, it sets the stage for injury.

I encourage many of my clients to visit a physical therapist for a full body evaluation and to get specific stretching and strengthening instruction to balance their muscles, so they can avoid getting hurt when they start being more active. Not every doctor will prescribe this, but if yours does or you have access to physical therapists who are in a private practice, I highly encourage you get a full evaluation. The evaluation can be eye-opening if the therapist explains where your strengths and weaknesses are and why the imbalances you have could cause an injury. It is often worth paying for yourself if your insurance doesn't cover the evaluation.

Another way to gain clarity from your body is by noticing the color of your urine. If you notice it is more yellow than it is clear, this is generally an indication you aren't getting enough hydration and need to drink more water. When you are dehydrated you will experience fatigue and a loss of coordination that can become serious. It is easy enough to drink water before and after you are aerobic, and it is best to have water with you whenever you are active.

Clarity also comes by paying attention to what is going on in your head. Be conscious of when you push yourself or when you disregard your pain, and notice what you are either feeling or thinking. Do the *"I am feeling … or I am thinking … because…"* inquiry and see what is driving your behavior. Do you think you should be doing something a certain way, because that is what you were told in the past or what you read? The inclusion of the word "should" in your self-talk can alert you to the possibility you are not paying attention to what your body is telling you or to what feels good or instinctively right. You want to feel good. If you don't feel good, understand why that is.

If you are avoiding aerobic activity or beating yourself up for not doing it, don't judge yourself. Focus on understanding what your real challenge is and what you can learn from the experience. Find an ah-ha insight out of the disappointment in missing your goals, and give yourself a chance to make changes or slight adjustments. Was the reason you didn't exercise a result of anxiety, boredom, your schedule, lack of planning, not looking forward to it or hating it, or was there another equally valid reason?

Only by seeing what is getting in your way of reaching your goal, can you start to look at how to address the problem. Maybe you really don't like the type of activity you are doing. If so, that is good to know, and this explanation gives you permission to finding something different you like more. Maybe you set an unrealistic goal, and now you can see you need to set goals each week that are more realistic. You don't have to set the same goal every week; that creates rigidity and a false expectation. It is often better to create fresh goals each week that are more realistic and based on what you really think you can achieve with complete confidence.

Madeline had a goal of being active five days a week, but she didn't always have control over her time. The fall we worked together, her daughters were going off to college and she had to pack up their things and drive them out of state. She was also going through a divorce and her mother in Florida needed her to go down periodically to help out. Most weeks she was pulled in different directions and some weeks were all her own. She set her goals accordingly, and if she got extra time to add in a walk or get to the gym that was a bonus.

A common problem many people have in meeting their goals is a lack of planning and preparation. If you don't have the right clothes with you on the day you planned to go for a bike ride, or if you frequently run out of time to fit in your activity, you may need help with better preparation. Observe and learn from the times when you can't do as you planned because you didn't have the time or didn't prepare what you needed. Then consider what would help you be more prepared. What do you need to do ahead of time? What changes in your schedule do you need to make and when do you need to make them? Perhaps a buddy would help provide some accountability. Anything that gets in the way of reaching your goals is a valid challenge. By seeing your challenges objectively, instead of judging yourself for your failures, you have a better chance of finding solutions.

Another form of clarity is having more information about how your body is impacted by your activity. It is worthwhile to spend some time learning about metabolism, aerobic conditioning, muscle flexibility and strengthening exercises.

Choices without Deprivation or a Need for Perfection

The fastest way to get derailed from being regularly active is doing something you hate. There is nothing worse or more de-motivating than dreading something and then beating yourself up for not doing it. The second week I worked with Gabriella, she was ready to throw in the towel. She said, "I can't do this. I didn't bike as I said I would, and I don't think this is going to work." I helped her see that she had succeeded by doing some biking, and we could easily revise her goal by picking a different activity so she had a greater chance of complete success. She chose walking and a strengthening program. Three years later, she is still doing these along with other aerobic activities.

Every January, millions of people join the gym and set high expectations of going no less than four times a week and sweating it out for at least thirty minutes. Two or three weeks later they quit out of disgust with themselves. They couldn't do it, couldn't maintain it, and couldn't stomach the thought of facing the gym one more time. The likelihood these people will join the gym again any time soon is nil. You may be one of them.

A bad experience doesn't mean you can't grow to love something that initially you aren't fond of doing. I certainly didn't enjoy the StairMaster when I first started using it, but I grew to like it within a couple of months and knew it would work for me. If you have limited options because of your weight or a physical handicap, you may also find it is worth doing one of those options, such as swimming, even if you aren't fond of it, so you can improve your abilities enough to move on to what you do enjoy more. Very often, when you first start exercising you find most everything seems a bit challenging. But if you really dislike an activity, and you don't find a way to enjoy it or to move on to something better, the likelihood you will stick with regular exercise is low.

Finding Your Motivation

A new behavior begins with having enough motivation to move out of your comfort zone and to encourage yourself to do something that doesn't come naturally in your daily routine. For some people, the motivation comes as a wake-up call that propels them into action, as it was for me. For others, they are motivated by a nagging voice that keeps rearing its head and finally gets loud enough it can no longer be avoided. And sometimes motivation occurs when you find yourself saying yes to an opportunity, such as a charity walk or an active vacation. In each case there is a defining moment when you are resolved to take action.

More often than not, the driving force — or catalyst — to get moving regularly is often to avoid the fate of something worse. What is worse can be weight gain, going on medication, the risk of disease, stress symptoms, fear of aging, not liking how you feel or look, or being criticized for not taking action. Fearing what you don't want to experience is often the catalyst that moves you from passive indifference to actively planning a change and then taking action. What you may not realize is a catalyst is a short-term motivator and doesn't keep you motivated when the going gets tough to stick with your new changes. The catalyst keeps you focused on what you don't want, rather than what you do want and what you are willing to work for to achieve it.

For Charise, who shared her story on my radio show, the catalyst was the fear of getting diabetes from watching the suffering her grandmothers went through, working in the healthcare field and taking a magazine survey that showed she was at high risk for the disease. These experiences added up, and the harsh reality scared her into action. But the disease isn't what she focused on. She got excited about taking control of her health and weight after reading up on living a healthier lifestyle, and she was motivated to exercise and eat better from learning about fitness, taking care of herself and gaining greater confidence in her abilities.

A catalyst motivator focuses on the negative, which is not enough to jazz you or give you inspiration to hold on to during the drudgery phases of change. To succeed, you have to have a positive outcome that matters to you, so you can go the distance and see yourself succeeding. An inspiring outcome is a different type of motivator and one that focuses on achieving well-being and feeling good. For me, the inspiration — or the prize — was to get back into my wardrobe of beautiful clothes, regain my health and feel good about myself. These were the long-term "feel good" motivators that overrode my internal whining about having to exercise and helped me stay on course for the two years it took to reach my goals. It was this longer term vision of what really mattered to me that got me into my sneakers and shorts most days of the week. And even when I lost sight of my vision, part of me remembered it so that I could sternly but gently ward off the resistance by telling myself, "No option"; "No discussion" and "Too bad girl, just go do it." And I did. I did it by keeping my eye on the prize, not by beating myself up with shoulds or focusing on what I didn't want.

Had I focused on losing weight, I would have given up in frustration. It took five months of being aerobic five or more days a week, eating healthier and reducing my stress before I saw any change in my weight. And then it seemed like I lost a whole dress size overnight. For the following four months, I seemed to plateau again before I lost another size one day, almost like magic. And again, I dropped another size one morning four months after the last time. During the first five months, when I didn't see any changes, it bothered me, but I hung in there. The second and third time I waited for a change, I was much more focused on other motivators that kept me going day-to-day and week-to-week. These motivators were reaching my daily and weekly aerobic activity goals, seeing myself achieve more endurance and strength, and feeling more alert, upbeat, confident, energized and productive. I felt good, even though my weight and how I fit in my clothes didn't change for months at a time. And when I did see a change, I felt excited and proud of myself. I had stuck with my routine long enough to see that I could reach my long term-goal.

Everyone is different in the way they lose weight, yet those that have done excessive dieting or experienced yo-yo weight loss as I have, will likely have plateaus when nothing seems to happen for long periods of time. Yet internally, healthy changes are happening to your body chemistry and metabolism you can't see. Isn't it reassuring to know that just because it doesn't seem like anything is happening, it really is, and there is nothing wrong with you if it takes some time? We don't all lose weight the same way or at the same pace, so if a friend of yours seems to be having more success than you, don't judge her for being better or you for being worse. Instead hang in there and be patient, as tough as that feels at the time. Once you reach your goal, you will have more than a slimmer body. You will have confidence that you can maintain it. And the time it took you to reach the goal will become a distant memory. I know, because those two years of perseverance paid off, and I've been wearing my clothes and staying in the best shape of my life ever since. It was so worth the effort during those months when I saw no results.

But unseen changes are hard to appreciate or understand. What many of my clients hope for when they first call me is immediate weight loss. "I want help losing weight," is usually the first thing out of their mouth. When I press them further, they also say they want to be fit, improve their health and feel better. I explain to them that in the first few months they may not lose any weight but instead will see improvements in their health, fitness level and well-being. The reason is that a lifestyle approach is not a quick-fix extreme weight loss method. Instead, weight loss and fitness is the natural outcome of a lifestyle based on healthier behaviors.

Even with healthier behaviors, not everyone will experience much weight loss. Gabriella, who is now seventy, would have liked to lose a bit of weight but has instead been very happy with her fitness and endurance results. She isn't much over weight, has been about the same size most of her life, and is at a stage where it is more difficult to significantly change her metabolism without doing an extreme regimen. So a minimal change in her weight is to be expected. She knows she wouldn't want or be able to do an extreme program, and she is happy doing what she can at an easier pace to improve her quality of life and feeling her best, which in the end is what really matters.

This lifestyle approach is a realistic process that works by helping you change your thinking and helping your body naturally and more easily recover from hormonal imbalances and a lowered metabolic rate. It takes time for your metabolism to move up and burn at a higher rate, and while you can force it to go up faster, you have greater success raising it more gently and slowly. Your metabolic rate is what determines your weight loss and your ability to lose the weight that matters most, which is fat weight. So while this is happening silently beneath the surface, watch for the other signs of progress. Feeling better and seeing yourself meet your activity goals and then progressing to doing more are those signs, and these signs are motivating in themselves.

Identifying What Really Motivates You

You are reading this book for a reason, so you probably have a problem you want to address or an issue you don't want to live with anymore. Whether that is motivating enough to get you to take action is another matter. What is important is to start acknowledging what concerns are starting to add up that you are no longer comfortable about, and what it is you really want to experience in your life.

Coaching Questions to

FIND YOUR MOTIVATION

Catalyst Motivators

What has scared or upset you about your health, fitness or weight in the past year?

Did any of these concerns ever motivate you to consider making a change?

What stopped you from making a change?

What would it take to be motivated to take action now?

What motivated you to start being more active in the past?

What do you notice about the times you are motivated to make changes?

Are there some types of situations that work as catalysts and others that you ignore?

Feel Good Motivators

How do you want to feel when you reach your goal?

What will you be able to do or be when you are more fit and healthy?

Why does this matter to you?

What are things you can do to remind yourself of what you want to achieve?

On a scale of 0 – 10, how motivated are you to start being more active or exercising now? (0 being not motivated, 10 being highly motivated)

If you are under a 7, what can you do to feel more motivated?

Getting Started

Are you now motivated to get started? Sometimes even when you don't have a motivating catalyst, the act of just starting anyway can take its place. Before you know it, you are moving and focusing on feeling good. Being ready to start is one thing. Knowing how to get started can be another, yet getting started is easier than you might think.

The best place to start is with some type of aerobic activity that gets you moving and feeling energized. While many experts encourage a mix of cardiovascular and strengthening exercises, both can be overwhelming when you first start and more of a commitment than most people can do when they begin. It is better to start with cardiovascular activities, which has both health and fitness benefits. After you build aerobic activity into your routine on a consistent basis, then you can more successfully add strengthening when you are ready to do more.

Setting Goals Loosely at First

Most programs recommend measuring and weighing yourself before you start and then getting on the scale weekly or even daily as part of setting your goals. Weighing yourself is the one thing I don't recommend. You already know if you are overweight and whether your weight is considerable or not. You don't need to measure yourself to know how you fit in your clothes or to feel any more distressed by your size.

When you rely on the scale as a measurement of your progress and success, it starts to have power over your motivation, emotions and behavior. And weighing yourself will become de-motivating if you don't see results as fast as you think you should, and very likely you won't. You will lose weight more slowly and will keep it off more successfully as an extension of your healthier behaviors. This weight loss approach may challenge your belief system if you've been conditioned to believe that faster weight loss is better. I suggest you don't use your scale, so you can avoid reinforcing your old beliefs or become so disillusioned you quit before making any real progress.

On the other hand, if you think it would be fun to have a before and later (note I didn't say after because with a lifestyle approach there is no after) set of measurements then feel free to do this once. Then put it away and focus on what really matters, which is becoming more active and fit so you feel better inside and out.

The first week of being active is a time to see what you are capable of doing. Your first week is not the time to set explicit goals or try to outdo yourself. Just set a goal of doing something aerobic a certain number of times that week. You don't want to be any more specific than that, and you don't want to push yourself at all. For example, if you haven't exercised or been active in a while, start off easy with a goal of being active on two days of the upcoming week for about ten or fifteen minutes. You don't even have to set a goal for how long you will be active. Then see how you do, how long you chose to be active, and how you feel.

Now you have information about what went well or didn't go so well to set goals for the following week. Set your new goals based on the number of days you can realistically fit in activity and for how long you can comfortably do it. The idea is to ease into exercising and activity by taking it easy, experimenting and learning from the challenges arise. More importantly, you want to set goals that you can succeed. If you set goals that are too difficult, you will set yourself up to fail at a time when you are still susceptible to your inner critic.

You may also want to check in with your doctor if you are on medications or at risk for heart disease to see if there is anything specific you should know, or to get a clearance for exercise, before getting too active.

Tracking Yourself

It will help you to have a way to track what you are doing so you can gauge your progress, be accountable to yourself and become conscious of how you are feeling and doing. The best way to do this is to create a fitness journal you can fill out easily for the week or for the month. There is no one right way to do this, and you may find that what you originally start with doesn't work for you and has to be adjusted.

You may also find that the idea of keeping a journal produces some anxiety and you don't want to write down what you are doing. This anxiety or resistance is worth investigating. Become curious about the feelings or thoughts you are having about keeping a fitness journal? See what past experience or belief these reactions are tied to, and then read on to see if what I am proposing offers a way where the journal can be beneficial and flexible enough to meet your current situation and needs. If you still decide you don't want to use one, let that be okay and see how well you stay on track without it. Then when you've been active for awhile, come back to the idea of keeping a journal or log. A fitness journal is very helpful if you are open to using it.

I suggest you create your own journal format based on the information that is important to you. You probably want to track the day of the week and the date, and you will want a place to put your goals and what you actually did. It also helps to have a place to write some comments about what happened, how you felt or even what didn't happen and why — to help you gain understanding (the second C: clarity) of what is getting in your way when you don't end up meeting all your goals. You may find there is a pattern when you look back at several weeks or months of journals.

Then you will probably want to track specific aspects of your fitness activities. If you decide to wear an activity monitor that tracks the calories burned or the steps taken when you are aerobically active, then create room in your journal for that. You will likely do more than one type of activity, which is important for variety and cross-training (more on cross-training later in this section), so you will want to record that. It also helps to track how many minutes you did, as well as your level of aerobic intensity, which I will also explain later in this section. And it can be useful to note any stretching you did. If you are strength training or doing any other non-aerobic activities, you probably will want other places in your journal for those entries.

Here's one type of journal (page 88) that many of my clients use. It includes many of the different items mentioned above. At the beginning of the week, or which ever day of the week you like to start with, write in the days and dates. Then put down the goals for the week.

On the first week, only write down the type of activity you want to do and on which days you think you will do them. It is fine if you actually do them on a different day, but this will help you think about when might be the best days and times and help you to start planning. It also helps you to be realistic about when you could really take the time, which minimizes setting yourself up with a goal you can't possibly meet.

This example from Sarah for her first week shows three goals to walk or bike on three days, so her goal is to be aerobically active three times this week. Any more than this would have been too much for her.

			Type of Activity	Minutes	Intensity	Calories Burned	Steps Taken	Stretches	Yoga
DAY	DATE								
M	2-6	GOAL	Walk						
		ACTUAL							
		COMMENT							
T	2-7	GOAL							
		ACTUAL							
		COMMENT							
W	2-8	GOAL	Bike						
		ACTUAL							
		COMMENT							
TH	2-9	GOAL							
		ACTUAL							
		COMMENT							
F	2-10	GOAL							
		ACTUAL							
		COMMENT							
S	2-11	GOAL	Walk						
		ACTUAL							
		COMMENT							
S	2-12	GOAL							
		ACTUAL							
		COMMENT							
		TOTALS							

During the week, Sarah filled in her journal with what she actually did and the total number of minutes she completed. Her comments helped her have greater awareness about how the activity felt and what made it challenging to be active one day yet fairly easy the next, which helped her understand how to set goals that were going to work better for her. Notice she biked a bit more than she felt comfortable and she was sore the next day. As you can see, she was starting to pay attention to the signals her body was sending her.

DAY	DATE		Type of Activity	Minutes	Intensity	Calories Burned	Steps Taken	Stretches	Yoga
M	2-6	GOAL	Walk						
		ACTUAL	Walk	20					
		COMMENT	This felt great and it was good to do during my lunch break.						
T	2-7	GOAL							
		ACTUAL							
		COMMENT							
W	2-8	GOAL	Bike						
		ACTUAL							
		COMMENT	I thought I could do this when I got home, but my meeting ran later than I expected it to.						
TH	2-9	GOAL							
		ACTUAL	Bike	15					
		COMMENT	I did this before dinner. It was tougher than I expected, but I did it.						
F	2-10	GOAL							
		ACTUAL							
		COMMENT	I feel a bit sore today.						
S	2-11	GOAL	Walk						
		ACTUAL	Walk	30					
		COMMENT	I felt fine today, and I walked a bit further than I planned but I felt good doing it.						
S	2-12	GOAL							
		ACTUAL							
		COMMENT	I didn't feel stiff or sore.						
		TOTALS		65					

Learning from What Went Well and What Didn't

What Sarah learned from the first week was she could walk twenty to thirty minutes and that it felt good, but that biking didn't feel good to her and she actually didn't like it all that much. She realized that just because she had a bike didn't mean she had to ride it. So she decided to try something that sounded a lot more appealing to her. She had some Richard Simmons aerobic videos she remembered using years before, and she remembered that she had fun doing them. So she decided for the second week to put down a goal of trying one of the tapes.

The second week, she not only listed the type of activity she was planning to do but also how long she would do them as her goals. She chose to set a goal of thirty minutes for both her walks because she knew that was realistic and enjoyable. She only chose twenty minutes for the video because she wasn't sure she could do it for a full half-hour. This was a smart decision and didn't push her beyond her capabilities or set herself up to be disappointed.

DAY	DATE		Type of Activity	Minutes	Intensity	Calories Burned	Steps Taken	Stretches	Yoga
		GOAL	Walk	30					
		ACTUAL							
M	2-13	COMMENT							
		GOAL							
		ACTUAL							
T	2-14	COMMENT							
		GOAL							
		ACTUAL							
W	2-15	COMMENT							
		GOAL	Richard Simmons video	20					
		ACTUAL							
TH	2-16	COMMENT							
		GOAL							
		ACTUAL							
F	2-17	COMMENT							
		GOAL	Walk	30					
		ACTUAL							
S	2-18	COMMENT							
		GOAL							
		ACTUAL							
S	2-19	COMMENT							
		TOTALS							

Be aware, that a goal for just five minutes is also alright when you are just starting a new type of activity, which is what Gabriella did when she first started using the elliptical machine at her gym. I remember the first time I got on my StairMaster; I thought I was going to die trying to do ten minutes and stopped at six minutes.

It is also fine to aim for five or ten minutes if you find walking a struggle and you are just starting to move after being sedentary for a long time. There is no judgment about how long is long enough. There are no comparisons to other people or any shoulds about how much you should be doing. That you are starting to move, experimenting with new things and giving yourself a chance is fantastic.

For those that can do more, great. But again don't compete with yourself — not yet anyway. Start off seeing what your body can do and pay attention to any warning signs. Those that think they are in as good a shape as they were ten or fifteen years ago, are the ones that get injured the fastest. Don't be a weekend warrior, or you may get sidelined for months. It isn't worth it. Give yourself a chance to ease into your new routine and then safely progress from there, as I will explain shortly.

At this point you may be having some resistance to setting goals. If so, be curious as to why that is and what you can do to change your perspective about goals. How can you do this in a way that works for you? If you don't see how to do this, then try being active for a few weeks without any goals and see what happens. Most likely within a few weeks you will want goals, and that is when you will begin to add them.

Understanding Aerobic Fitness

The objective for being more active or exercising is to increase your aerobic fitness, which reduces the risk of heart disease, improves insulin sensitivity and blood sugar levels, relieves anxiety and depression and amps up energy. Easy walks or bike rides for fifteen minutes a couple of times a day will help you achieve these benefits. If you aren't active enough to get your heart rate up into the fat-burning zone or if you pick an activity that doesn't keep you consistently moving, be aware you won't see the changes in your physique that you are probably looking for.

To burn fat (as well as carbohydrates), you need to move continually with enough intensity – or exertion – to get your heart rate between 60 to 85 percent of your maximum heart rate. To get the other benefits I mentioned in the preceding paragraph, you only need to exert yourself enough to get your heart rate above 50 percent of its maximum. When you exceed 85 percent of your heart rate maximum, you will burn carbohydrates faster and build greater aerobic fitness, but you will no longer be burning fat. The reason has to do with the way the aerobic system works in the body. When you are aerobic, the oxygenated blood pumped by your heart out to your muscles provides the oxygen necessary to convert fat and carbohydrates into energy. Fat is not converted without enough oxygen. This is why you've heard that when you are aerobic you burn fat and carbohydrates, and the more aerobic you are the more fat and carbohydrates you will burn.

However there is a limit to how much more exertion you want to do. When you are exerting yourself so much that you can't talk, you are hyperventilating and your heart can't pump the blood fast enough to provide enough oxygen needed for the creation of aerobic energy. At that point the body shifts to producing anaerobic energy, which doesn't rely on oxygen. Anaerobic energy also doesn't use fat as a source of fuel, only carbohydrates. So when you hear the terms fat-burning zone and anaerobic threshold, it means that you want to stay primarily in the fat-burning zone and only cross the anaerobic threshold (going over 85 percent of your maximum heart rate) when doing interval training. I will address more about interval training in a bit.

Knowing Your Aerobic Levels

The formula for finding your maximum heart rate (MHR) is:

220 − (your age) = _____ beats per minute (pbm)

For example if you are 50, the formula for your MHR would be:

220 − 50 = 170 bpm

From this you can multiply your MHR by 60% and 85% to get your range.

_____pbm x .65 = _____pbm   _____pbm x .85 = _____pbm

Using our example of 170 as the max heart rate (MHR), that would be:

170 bpm x .65 = 111 bpm   170 pbm x .85 = 145 pbm

This means for someone who is 50, their fat-burning zone is between 111 and 145 bpm.

Note: This is a generic formula and may not fit everyone perfectly, and it is not applicable to those people taking beta blockers.

Once you know your fat-burning range, there are several ways to determine what your heart rate actually is when you are active. The easiest is to get a good heart rate monitor and wear it when you are moving. Another is to use equipment that has a heart rate monitor built in and hold onto the hand grips to get a reading. And the third is to do the talk test and pay attention to what you perceive your exertion levels to be.

This last option is actually very easy and a great way to be more conscious of your body and how you are feeling. It is called the Rate of Perceived Exertion (RPE). You can perceive how hard you are working and how that translates into your heart rate level by how easy or hard it is to talk for at least one full minute, as you see in this graphic.

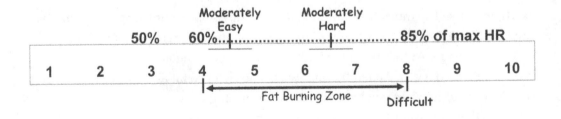

2-3	Easy	Can talk with no problem – feels easy
4-5	Moderately Easy	Talking is still fairly easy – feeling bit of exertion
6-7	Moderately Hard	Talking takes more effort – feeling like some work
8	Difficult	Can't keep up a conversation – feeling like hard work
9-10	Extremely Difficult	Can't really talk at all

Note: Be sure to test this for at least one full minute to see what your exertion level really is. If you test it using less time, you may think you can talk fairly easily. The question is, can you keep on talking for the full minute just as easily?

Choosing Moderate Intensities

The fat-burning zone is primarily a moderate level of exertion — from moderately easy to moderately hard. It always surprises people when they discover the fat-burning zone is much less work than they expected and can seem almost too easy, which it would seem if you've been accustomed to working as hard as you can to build up a sweat and feel the burn. Feeling the burn by the way is a sign that you are exercising in the anaerobic zone and experiencing a build up of lactic acid in your muscles. Lactic acid isn't a problem, but it does indicate physical stress, which people who are athletes are better conditioned to handle.

Suffice it to say that when you get started, especially if you haven't been active in a while or you suffer from arthritis, have diabetes or are very overweight, your objective is to be aerobic within the lower end of the fat-burning zone and to work your way up in exertion from moderately easy to moderate. Those who are obese have to be particularly careful to avoid moving too fast or too hard in order to protect themselves from extra force on the body, which can lead to stress fractures, tendon strains or a higher risk of osteoarthritis. As those people with extra weight get stronger, lighter and healthier, they can move faster and move up to more moderately hard levels.

It is best to mix up the level of intensities, instead of always moving at the same pace. Our bodies adapt quickly to our routines, and if we don't mix them up we will plateau at the same level of results for longer periods of time. This may partially explain why I plateaued for months at a time when I used my StairMaster for the first two years. I did the same program for the same amount of time the same number of days a week for months on end. That is not the best way to get results.

In addition, new research indicates that low to moderate intensity exercise has greater impact on reducing LDL (bad) cholesterol than higher intensity activity, and the reverse is true for improving HDL (good) cholesterol. Higher intensity exercise appears to increase HDL as compared to lower exertion rates. So clearly a mix of the two intensities is beneficial, but if you can only move at a slower pace you are still getting significant benefit and soon enough you will be able to increase your rate of exertion.

The very best way to get results is to mix up the amount of time you are active, your intensity levels and the types of things you do during the week. This is why it is important to have at least two different types of activities in your routine, which is called cross-training. You want to spice things up and keep your body guessing or it will adapt to what you are doing and slow down the progress in reaching your goals. You don't want that. You will also find this keeps things much more interesting.

Selecting Aerobic Activities

Now that you understand a bit more about aerobic fitness, you can select any activity that gets your heart rate up into the fat-burning zone and keeps you moving. When you think of it in these terms, there are many more options than you probably thought.

If you love to be outdoors you might consider kayaking, canoeing, wind surfing, hiking, cross-country skiing, snow shoeing, broom ball, ice skating, roller blading, biking, walking, Nordic walking or running. Outdoor boot camps can be exhilarating and so can preparing for a race or triathlon. If you like team sports see if there are local places you can play softball, basketball, ice hockey, racquet ball, tennis or golf. And for light activities, you can do gardening or Tai Chi, a moving meditation practice that originated in China as a martial art.

For those who prefer to be indoors or need a place to go during the winter months, think what would be the most enjoyable. You can choose from activities such as dancing, aerobics classes, exercise videos, power yoga, water aerobics, swimming, rowing, kickboxing, Pilates, yoga, Tai Chi, fitness classes and using exercise equipment. See the full list of activities in the appendix for other ideas to start a new aerobic activity.

Melanie knew exactly what she wanted to start with. She used to do contra dancing, which is a type of New England folk dancing that is a bit like square dancing. It had been years since she last square danced, but she knew of a group that gathered at a local church once a week nearby and she decided it would be a fun way to be aerobic. She had also just gotten her kids a Wii (Nintendo interactive video game) that came with a sports package, including interactive bowling. She used to love bowling as a teen, and she was having a blast showing her kids how it was done. Wii and other interactive fitness games (Dance Dance Revoluion, PlayStation2 and XBox) are a lot of fun and a great way to involve friends or the whole family.

As Melanie learned, you may rediscover types of aerobic activities that you once enjoyed when you were younger. Maybe you once loved using the hula hoop like the gal I met at the diabetes conference, or maybe you used to enjoy roller blading, ice skating, cross-country skiing or swing dancing. Why not take them up again?

Planning & Preparation

Some activities you can do by just walking out your door or clearing a spot in front of your TV, others require a bit more planning and preparation. If you don't have good footwear, get some. This will minimize discomfort and the potential for injury. If you need to have clothes with you at work or in the car, figure out the best way to plan for this. If you won't be going home afterward, be sure to pack some food because you will probably be hungry when you are done. And always carry water with you, and if at all possible do so in a non-plastic bottle. We are starting to learn that toxins get leached from the plastic into your water, particularly if the bottles get heated up and that can happen in your car.

Coaching Questions to
GET STARTED

What types of aerobic activities to you think you would like to do and that you can do?   (See a list of activities in the appendix on page 213.)

What do you need to do to be prepared on the days you plan to be active?

What will work best for you to track your exertion level?

What else do you need to get started?

Keeping Yourself on Track

The first few months of starting to be more active is also a time when you can easily get derailed. For most people the first week or two feels easy, but soon after that it feels like work. It is work to change your behaviors because we are creatures of habit and gravitate to what feels better at the time — even if we know choosing to avoid activity won't really feel better later.

Pick things you enjoy doing, have a reason for doing it that trumps your resistance, and arm yourself with whatever it takes to keep you motivated day-to-day and week-to-week.

It will take several months before your new lifestyle changes are a natural part of your weekly routine, and the pull of what is more comfortable, familiar and easier will require you to find ways to stay on track. Some days you won't be able to overcome your inner voice that says, "I can't do it now" or "I don't want to do this." You may find yourself slipping back into your sedentary habits without even realizing it or you may do it knowingly and with a mental stick that makes you feel so badly you don't want to face the pain it causes.

The most important thing you can do to stay on track is to give yourself permission not to be perfect. You won't always make your weekly or daily goal. No one does, with the exception of people in training. So give up the idea that you must be good to be on track. Instead, focus on what you actually can do, push yourself through the times you resist, learn from what gets in the way, and remember that as the days and weeks add up that missing a day or two here and there doesn't much matter.

What matters is giving yourself room to be imperfect and understanding that the journey isn't a smooth straight path of starting on day one and reaching the end goal on day ninety without mishaps. It is instead a process of ups and downs in which life and your attitude will get in the way, and from these experiences you will learn more about yourself and how to get past these challenges and move on.

Remembering Why You Care

Feeling motivated is the key to sticking with something that feels difficult, so it helps to find ways to remind yourself of the end goal and why you really care about being fit and healthy in the first place. You answered the questions earlier in this section, so you do know or have a good idea of why it matters to you, but on a daily basis you may forget or it may feel too removed from your current reality to motivate you. To help you remember and keep it fresh in your mind, find things that represent your vision. Ideally these will feel both inspiring and good when you see or hear them.

There are many different ways to do this. Some people create collages of pictures and images that represent what they see themselves doing when they are fit. For example, you can use pictures of people hiking, skiing, playing with grandchildren, gardening, tennis, speaking or whatever it is that you want to experience in your life. Some of my clients keep pictures of their kids out, to remind them they are getting fit to be healthy enough to be there for their kids. Others use pictures of themselves when they were in better shape. One client used a picture of a relative who was sickly as a reminder of what she didn't want to have happen to her, and while this was an image of what she didn't want, it provided an image in her mind of what she did want, which worked.

I hung up a few pictures and read stories of fit women from magazines that were realistic for me. It doesn't help to find women who look perfect because that is unrealistic for most of us, and if you don't believe it is realistic for you, it won't help. Every month, the major fitness and women's health magazines feature two or three success stories about real women just like you, who used a lifestyle approach to get healthy and slim down. Most are happy to be a size 10, 12 or 16, because they learned that it wasn't how much weight they lost but how good they felt that truly mattered in the end.

What else might work for you? Maybe something like sea shells is more symbolic of what you want to feel or do, and you could put the shells in conspicuous places as reminders. Or perhaps you are more motivated by hanging an outfit you eventually want to wear again in a place where you can see it regularly. I used to stand in my closet and picture myself wearing all my great clothes, and it wasn't hard to do because I had worn them before. I could see myself in my tan slacks feeling confident or in my pink dress feeling sexy. You too have things you can remember feeling good in.

The catch 22 is not getting attached to whether you actually get back in those clothes. It is the feeling you want, and yes you would love to wear those clothes again, but sometimes you don't control the actual outcome. Our bodies can't be forced to become and stay a certain size, and for some it is not possible to get back into those smaller sizes. After years of dieting, dealing with hormonal changes and aging, your natural healthy body size and weight may be something different than you expect. But as you will find, once you start taking care of yourself, feeling better, getting fit and gaining confidence, you will come to appreciate your body at the place that feels best — and that isn't based on a size or what is on the scale.

Figuring Out What Motivates You Week-to-Week

Knowing what motivates you to be active for the long-term is only half the battle. The other half is being motivated by more immediate goals than a longer term vision. Everyone is different in what motivates them week-to-week, and you may have to experiment to see what actually inspires you to stay moving.

Some people are motivated by reaching a specific target achievement, training for a specific event, or mastering something. Others are motivated by completing daily goals and checking things off. And there are many who are motivated when they compete with themselves or others. You may not know which of these will keep you motivated, so you could try a few things and see if they hold your interest. If not, try something else. It is fine to decide that what you thought would be motivating wasn't and to stop doing it and try something else.

I've found people are either motivated by reaching their daily or weekly goals, or by reaching a specific goal that is attainable within about three months. You want to see results soon enough that you won't give up. This is why many fitness and coaching programs are about twelve weeks long and include daily or weekly goals. Three months isn't so long you can't see light at the end of the tunnel, yet it is long enough to experience weekly progress and some significant changes. This serves both types of people.

Picking an Accomplishment to Work Toward
Those who are motivated by an end goal do well picking things they want to accomplish or be fit enough to do by a certain date, like being able to walk for thirty minutes four times a week, swim a mile, or participate in a charity event, race, or hiking vacation in three months.

Savannah surprised herself by how motivated she became knowing she was going to participate in a two-day walk for cancer. She spent months walking nearly every day in a local park or at the beach to build up her stamina and endurance, and she was proud to complete the walk with the other women on her team. As she prepared for the big event, she discovered how much better she felt and how much she valued the time she spent connecting with herself on those long and peaceful walks. When it was over, she celebrated her success and then kept up her routine.

Letting Go of the Weight Loss Goal
Many of my clients are not ready to pick an event or focus on a specific goal with the exception of weight loss. Some people are successful using the scale, but most aren't. Find out for yourself by being conscious of your behaviors after you weigh yourself. If you are reacting to what the scale says by changing your behaviors and having an emotional reaction, get it out of the house or only use it periodically. Don't let it run you. If you really want to have a weight loss goal for the twelve weeks, then make it just five pounds and don't penalize yourself if you don't fully achieve that goal or don't stop your new healthy behaviors if you exceed it.

Everyone who successfully achieves regular exercise or is regularly active will tell you that they stopped caring about their weight and came to focus instead on being healthy. I did the same thing. I weighed myself periodically during my first two years and have since tossed out the scale. I no longer care and really don't know what I weigh. I am not alone. More people are coming to realize the number of the scale is meaningless.

Kelly LeBrock, who succeeded in losing thirty-one pounds in the Celebrity Fit Club reality show, starved herself and exercised twice a day to reach that goal. Two years later she acknowledged in People magazine that this wasn't good for her and she is happier and healthier without weighing herself. She now accepts herself being heavier and curvier and so does her new husband.

Getting Pumped by Tracking What You've Done

Many of my clients tell me they love seeing what they've accomplished each week and almost as many like seeing this in numbers because it makes the accomplishment real to them. Numbers are something you can see and understand. This explains why so many people get attached to weighing themselves. They can see how they are doing relative to a number.

Instead of tracking your weight, you can select a more positive and empowering number relative to an activity you have done – as in tracking steps, calories burned, minutes, distance or intensity. These are numbers you have control over, and they help you set goals, see progress and keep you motivated day-to-day during the week. You can see what you have done and what you need to do to achieve your goals.

One of the best tools to help you track your progress is an accurate activity monitor. These can be pedometers that track your steps, calorie accelerometers that track how many calories you burn when you move, or pedometers that do both. There are many products on the market to choose from at many different price points, but if you focus only on price you will more likely get a product you can't rely on for accuracy. You will learn very quickly that numbers you can't trust are de-motivating and can lead you to give up on your goals. Instead pick a product that is highly reliable.

From my experience the best activity calorie tracker is the Caltrac, and it always gets five-star reviews. I wore mine for almost eighteen months when I first got it, and I loved it. After that I didn't need it for motivation. You can order it online from Wal-Mart for around $40 (2008 prices).

Another product that I've used with my clients is the NL series by New Lifestyles, which is a combination pedometer and accelerometer. These are a bit more expensive, but if you want accuracy and the option of steps or calories burned these are worth it. This company also makes a reliable pedometer. Accusplit is another company with good pedometers, and they certify the accuracy of their products.

Clarissa knew she liked using the pedometer the first week she tried it and found it motivating at the gym. She then wore it when she went on vacation and discovered that other aerobic activities, including biking, golf, tennis, walking and running, were as good as the exercising she did on equipment. In her mind, she only equated what she did at the gym with exercise. This was eye-opening for her, and she then wanted to mix things up more on the weekends, which would allow her to meet her goals while spending time with her husband and kids.

Clarissa chose to wear her pedometer while being active, but other clients like to wear their pedometer or calorie tracker all during the day. It validates they are being active, even if it isn't always aerobic, and it demonstrates the difference between inactive and active days. They can see for themselves they aren't burning as many calories on days they aren't being aerobic and active, and like Clarissa, they can see how much more they burn when they are aerobic. For Irene, the Caltrac drove home how much she needed to be aerobically active. She also found she preferred calorie tracking to steps, and found it more motivating.

Not everyone finds either of these motivating. Katie told me right from the beginning that she wouldn't be motivated by using an activity monitor. I still encouraged her to try it anyway because she might discover it would work for her, and she wouldn't know if she didn't try. I sent her a loaner Caltrac to try out, and she was surprised to learn that she did like it and wore it while being aerobic. Others found they disliked it as much as they thought and sent it back. I didn't pressure them either way. My goal wasn't to force them into using these devices or into what I thought was best.

It doesn't matter what motivates anyone else; what matters is what works for you and having the freedom to figure that out for yourself. Don't rule things out unless you know with certainty it won't work because you may surprise yourself and find the one thing that truly does keep you accountable to yourself.

Sarah was one who found that she liked seeing how many calories she burned and she only wanted to track this when she was being aerobic. As you can see in her weekly journal, she is recording her calories and discovering she burns more when she does her videos than when she walks. This information maps to her perceived rate of intensity and validates what she physically feels.

DAY	DATE		Type of Activity	Minutes	Intensity	Calories Burned	Steps Taken	Stretches	Yoga
		GOAL	Walk	40					
		ACTUAL	Walk	55	4-5	385		4	3
M	3-6	COMMENT	I was able to go a bit further today. It was beautiful out and I added an extra loop.						
		GOAL							
		ACTUAL							3
T	3-7	COMMENT							
		GOAL							
		ACTUAL							3
W	3-8	COMMENT							
		GOAL	Richard Simmons video	40					
		ACTUAL	Richard Simmons	40	6-7	388		5	3
TH	3-9	COMMENT	Still love this video						
		GOAL							
		ACTUAL	Walk	32	4-5	226		4	3
F	3-10	COMMENT	Did the walk today instead, because I will have to go to a meeting tomorrow night						
		GOAL	Walk	40					
		ACTUAL							
S	3-11	COMMENT							
		GOAL	Leslie Sansone video	40					
		ACTUAL	Leslie Sansone	35	5-8	326			3
S	3-12	COMMENT	I got her other 4 mile walk video that had some jogging in it. It was a bit tough, but ok.						
		TOTALS		162		1325			

A common mistake people make is to assume that only those activities that burn the most calories are the ones you should focus on. That reinforces the no-pain-no-gain belief, and it isn't true. It has been proven that it is best to have a mix of easy, moderate and hard days during the week, which not only keeps your body from adapting to one thing it also gives your body a chance to recover after doing more intense aerobic activity. Sarah has a good mix or varying levels of intensity, and they are all within the fat-burning zone.

Once she tracks her numbers for a few weeks, she will know how to set goals for calories burned and can begin setting weekly goals for this along with her goals for the number of minutes she wants to accomplish. Everyone burns calories at a different rate based on weight, height and age. So you can't make any assumptions about how much you should burn or compare yourself to anyone else. Instead you have to see what is true for you and then use that as a guideline for setting your goals.

Sarah is also keeping track of the number of stretches she does each day. On the days she is aerobically active, she does four additional types of stretches than on her non-active days. She does a series of three yoga postures each day, and when she is aerobic she adds in a stretch for her hamstrings, quadriceps, hips and calves for a total of seven different stretches.

You can also determine if you find it more motivating to set goals for each day or for the whole week. Many of my clients find it more helpful initially to do it by the day, knowing that there is flexibility as to which day they actually achieve the goal. The daily goals help them plan their week and be more realistic about what they can achieve. At some point, I've noticed, most eventually switch to setting weekly goals for the number of days and minutes they want to be aerobic and the number of days they want to do other routines. In Sarah's case that would be a total weekly goal of four days and 160 minutes of aerobic activity.

Letting Your Body Guide Your Progression

The fastest way to get off track and derailed is to get hurt or to feel overwhelmed, burned out, or sick and tired. Unfortunately, we as a society aren't conditioned to pay attention to what our bodies are trying to tell us. I have had several injuries since beginning to be active because I didn't pay attention to the warning signs. I didn't learn after the first incident because each type of pain is different, and I still didn't understand that any ache, sharp pain, snapping sensation or intuitive sense that something might be wrong was worth addressing. All I knew was to push through any discomfort because that is what I had been taught, and because I was focused on performance.

This determination to compete with myself and do what I thought I should be able to do has led to shoulder, calf and upper arm injuries. It is the same type of competitive determination that led to 9,000 reported yoga-related injuries between 2004 and 2005 according to the U.S. Consumer Product Safety Commission. Imagine how many more went unreported. My mother was one of those unreported statistics when she tore her meniscus when she went back to yoga after twenty years.

If you don't know how to let your body and inner wisdom guide you, the normal thing is to turn to someone else who is an expert to tell you what to do. And that is what everyone does, but this one-sided expertise doesn't work very well.

Many fitness experts will give you a set program that tells you the specific exercises, amount of time and level of effort you have to do. Such rigidity doesn't take into account what your body can really do or if you are ready to start at those levels. Instead the focus is on getting you up to speed as quickly as possible to reach rapid goals. This is particularly the case in boot camps and on reality shows.

It is true that personal trainers will conduct a fitness assessment before you work with them, and they do have a good idea of what your capabilities are. But their mindset is focused on the principles of exercise physiology, which emphasizes overloading your cardiovascular, muscular and skeleton systems. So they will start you off close to your limit and then see what more you can do. It is their job is to push you past your comfort zone so you get results, and that is fine when you are ready for that. Most who have been sedentary or who are obese aren't ready for it when they first start being aerobically active. I wasn't ready for a year, so I waited to work with a trainer until I had achieved a consistent cardio routine and built up my stamina.

Taking Advantage of What Trainers Have to Offer

Don't get me wrong, personal trainers can help you a great deal and I do encourage you to consider working with one when you have incorporated at least 120 minutes of cardio exercise into your weekly routine for an extended period of time. How long that period of time should be is up to you, but I would say at least a couple of months. By then you will be more fit and prepared to go into a gym or have a trainer come to your home, and you will by ready to learn a lot from him or her. Most importantly this professional can show you how to properly perform strengthening exercises, whether that is by using hand weights, elastic tubing, stability balls, medicine balls, weighted bars, circuit equipment, benches or any other equipment to which you or they have access.

Once you have a trainer, he or she can teach you other ways of overloading, which is actually the way you make progress. This may sound counter-intuitive to what I'm telling you in this book, but it isn't. Overloading is how you improve aerobic fitness, increase bone density, retain flexibility and develop stronger muscles. Very simply, when you overload your cardiovascular system with aerobic activity you improve your heart, lungs and vascular health. When you overload your bones with low-impact weight bearing exercise such as walking and dancing, you increase bone mass. When you stretch, you are elongating a shortened muscle for greater mobility. And when you overload your muscles with enough resistance from strengthening exercises, you build muscle mass.

Personal trainers can give you programs and introduce you to new types of exercises you can do with them or on your own. What you want to avoid is forming a dependency on a trainer to ensure you meet your goals. If you discover you are only motivated to show up because you are paying them and not being active or doing your other routines when they aren't around, you will know you are no longer in control and have a high chance of quitting when you stop working with your trainer. When this happens, you have stopped doing things for yourself and are only doing it because someone makes you.

It is better to work with a trainer when you're already committed enough to yourself that you willingly do your aerobic activity even when they aren't around. This way you can decide to work with a trainer for whatever length of time is best for you, taking from them what they have to offer and doing things on your own or by mixing it up with other instructors and trainers. If you settle in for the long run with one trainer, you may lose your power and your initiative. Again, you know yourself best and you have to make decisions that suit your goals and needs.

Recognizing Your Limits

There is a difference between overloading yourself within your limits and being pushed too far. Being pushed past your limit is a fast way to injury, over-exertion and giving up. If you've ever watched the reality fitness shows, you've seen how much work it is, how much is expected of them the first week and how often the contestants want to quit. Consider if what you see them doing would be motivating for you and if you would really be able to incorporate the new behaviors into your lifestyle after the program ends. If not, don't do it.

Also consider if it is safe. I watched the *Obesity Olympics* sponsored by 20/20 a number of years ago with alarm. Two families competed to lose the most weight. The parents and children were all clinically obese and close to three hundred pounds each. The first thing they had to do was run a mile. It was painful to watch because both families were clearly putting themselves through agony to comply and it put them at risk of suffering a heart attack or experiencing an injury. The next eight weeks they struggled through a grueling, high-intensity regime overseen by two Olympic athletes and their trainer. In the end each person lost close to twenty pounds. Was it worth it to put them through this? Did they choose to exercise or find a way to maintain their fitness afterward? Did they maintain their weight loss? This program was so extreme I doubt it.

Since then more people have participated on the *Biggest Loser*, the *Celebrity Fit Club*, *I Want to Look Like a Cheerleader Again*, and other fitness or weight loss reality shows. Some of these shows are more extreme than others, and some of the contestants are more prepared than others to handle the intensity and to maintain their changes when they go home.

If you decide it is worth pursuing a hard-core program, be sure to understand the risks and liability waivers. You will definitely get faster results and the accountability to keep you in line, but the results won't last if you don't follow up with a fitness lifestyle on your own when the program ends. Many of the contestants (including winners) on the *Biggest Loser* and *Celebrity Fit Club* haven't been able to maintain what they lost after the show ends. Some figure out a way to recreate their new fitness lifestyle once they are back in their normal surroundings, but many struggle to stick with the program on their own.

Knowing When to Take it Slow

What works better for most people is a process that starts off easy and is driven by what feels good, and that is determined by paying attention to your body. If you let your body be your guide, you will discover the more you do, the more you can do and want to do. You will get excited and motivated by the changes in yourself and want to see what else you can do.

When it gets easy to do something that once felt challenging, you will push yourself a little bit further. When you accomplish a small goal, you will set a slightly higher one. And if you can do that, you will want to see if you can do more. When you are driving the pace without comparing yourself to others or what you think you should do, you won't overdo it. Instead you will guide your progress with steady improvements to greater long term success. This approach is positive, reinforcing and confidence building.

When Anne first started walking on her treadmill she didn't think walking was really exercise and pushed herself to go as fast as she could. She struggled to keep up with the pace, and was surprised when she met with her trainer who told her to lower the pace way down to the point it felt she could keep up fairly easily. Not only did she learn the pace she had been doing was too fast for her and it was not only okay to go slower but recommended, she also learned walking absolutely is great aerobic exercise. Anne's experience immediately changed from dreading to loving her time on the treadmill because she could do it and she felt good about it. Soon she was building up her time and speed. Her confidence from walking motivated her to try strength training, which she discovered she enjoyed so much it became her passion and today she is an award-winning body-builder. She could never have imagined this when she first started walking.

Karen, another guest on my show, also started off setting very small goals for herself so she wouldn't get set up for a disappointment. She started with the treadmill and set the pace low enough she could walk for thirty minutes. Then she began to increase the incline and the speed a little bit each week as she got stronger. It took a year before she felt ready to take an aerobics class she wanted to do, and she was so glad she waited.

She was able to get through it and enjoy herself, and now it is a place she goes to be with new friends and to spice up her routine.

When I first started using my StairMaster I could do about ten minutes and within a month I was up to thirty minutes and then a month later forty-five minutes. It was then that I started to increase the intensity and went from level three to a four, and six months later I was at a level five. A year later I was easily doing level seven. My second year I added strength training to my routine because I was ready for it and found myself wanting it. It felt so good to see myself do more and get stronger. I loved how it felt and how I felt in my body.

One good guideline for progressing in aerobic fitness is to first focus on increasing the amount of time you spend, and when you reach thirty minutes consistently you can focus on making it more difficult. If you make it too difficult too soon, you won't be able to do more than about fifteen to twenty minutes and it will be nearly impossible to progress past that point.

Ellis was experiencing this limitation. He told me he road his Health Rider elliptical machine for about twenty minutes and couldn't do any more. When I asked him on a scale of 1-10 how hard he was riding it, he said about a level nine. He had trained hard in the military and anything less didn't seem hard enough, but I convinced him to slow down to a level five or six and see how that went. He found that much easier, and once his body had a chance to do this for few weeks for about thirty to four-five minutes and recover, I encouraged him to go back up a bit to levels between five and eight. Now he was more effective at burning fat, felt better and could get a longer aerobic session in. He also got better results.

Many of my clients start out thinking they have to aim for the high end of the exertion scale and are surprised when I encourage them to slow down, but they always feel better and notice they have less pain afterward. If you are ever getting pain or feel exhaustion, let this guide you to lesson your pace, take a day off and get more rest.

Gabriella had put her back out during a week when she was too sick to be very active, so she was nervous about going back to the gym even though she was feeling better and her back was improving. She knew moving would help her back, and she had already started walking and feeling some relief. I asked her what she thought would be best to do at the gym, and she said there were certain things she knew she wouldn't do like overhead raises and the leg curl machine and she wouldn't push herself on the elliptical. She was very clear what was not going to feel good to her, which were the things that wouldn't be good for her back. I also suggested she lighten the weights when she did her other strengthening exercises that week and to eliminate all the weight on those that involved her back so that she could focus just on mobility instead of strengthening. I also reminded her to stop doing anything that was even slightly painful.

What she was learning was how to take it easy after an injury, which eliminated the fear and allowed her to bounce back more quickly to what she was doing before her back went out. More importantly she was being reminded that she could trust her own instincts. She did know what was best because she had gotten very good at listening to her body and giving herself permission to take it easy and not push.

Establishing Realistic Routines

Creating a routine you can live with is a key factor in keeping yourself on track. Your routine will include what you do during your active fitness time, being prepared with the proper clothing and shoes, and finding times in your schedule you can consistently dedicate to your new routine.

<u>Making the Time</u>

If you are wondering when the best time to be active is, the answer is whenever you can find time to do it. There is however one time that isn't ideal and that is within an hour or two before going to bed, because you will be revving up your metabolism just as your body needs to turn it down for sleep. Other than that, any time that works for you is the best time.

Finding enough time can be challenging if you have a busy schedule and don't see a place to fit an activity into your day. Consider what things in your schedule can be moved up or back a bit, if you could slip away at some point during a lunch break or when the kids have something else going on. Everyone who has succeeded will tell you that the only way you will find time is if you make it, and that means making it a priority. Those who have a significant health scare and realize that without their health their quality of life suffers find the time. As I mentioned earlier, I now plan my day around it. It is that important to me.

Randee never thought she could be active more than about once or twice a week. But once she found she liked how it felt, she began to find the time. She got up a bit earlier to exercise and discovered she had extra time afterward for herself and she was meeting the day with a more positive attitude. Once she got a taste for how much better she could feel, she saw things differently and realized what she initially perceived as an obstacle really wasn't.

She also began to set aside about five minutes in the morning to schedule her day. She saw ways to couple errands together and make arrangements to be home in time to make a good dinner for her family. Her planning helped her to get to bed earlier so she could get enough sleep, which eliminated her chronic exhaustion. She admitted this took some time to put planning into her life and change her habits. But once she did it, it really worked. She came to understand that health was at the top of the list for her and her family, and it was central to everything else being built around it. Through her own planning and actions, her husband and daughters gradually made healthier choices and joined her in being more active and eating better.

Planning and Preparation

Planning and preparation is unavoidable if you want to succeed. There are things you need to do to be ready to exercise or be active. You need to make the time, have ways to remind yourself, have your clothing and anything else you need with you, eat a couple of hours earlier and then soon after you are done (particularly if you have hyper or hypoglycemia), and drink enough water.

"My challenge," said Renee when she was looking back at the week and understanding why she struggled to meet her goals, "is being prepared." She could see that if she didn't make arrangements with her family and have things prepared ahead of time that she couldn't get to the gym. She could also see that she was using her lack of preparation as an excuse, and she discovered the excuse was weighing her down and draining her energy. She loved the class at the gym, and her lack of being ready was upsetting her. Once she got a plan in place, the routine just flowed and she got energized by the class and the people she met there.

In some cases you also need to plan what you will be doing when you are doing your fitness routine, as in the case of strengthening exercises. You may need to get your equipment set up and then see what order you will be doing your routine in. It is a good idea to write down what you do each time so you can easily determine which weights or resistance levels to use and how to progress from one time to the next.

Adding in the Warm Up and Cool Down

If you are going to be active at fairly high levels of intensity (as in exceeding a 6 or 7 on the rate of perceived exertion scale) you will want to warm up your muscles and joints to reduce stiffness and avoid injury for five minutes or so before hand. Warming up is not the same as stretching. Warming up is getting limber and preparing your body to move by gently and rhythmically moving the parts of your body you will be using while being aerobically active or strengthening. For example, marching in place, rotating your shoulders and doing neck rolls before going for a jog or run. Afterward, stretching, such as a calf or hamstring stretch is done to loosen up the muscle and increase range of motion. This is best done after aerobic activity when muscles are warmed up from increased blood flow. It is not recommended to stretch prior to being active because stretching a cold muscle can lead to strains.

After you have completed a moderately hard or difficult session, give yourself another five minutes to gradually reduce your pace, instead of stopping cold. When you stop cold, you run the risk of having your blood pool up in your extremities and slowed circulation of blood back to your heart, brain and muscles. The cool down works to acclimate your heart rate, blood pressure and metabolism back to their normal state and will minimize muscle stiffness and dizziness. Cool downs are very important for those who have high blood pressure or are at risk for heart disease.

Checking in With Yourself

One of the keys to staying on track is taking time to check in and review your goals and accomplishments at the end of each week, whenever you decide that is. This is something you can do on your own or with someone that is supporting, training or coaching you.

Use your journal and add up your times and see how you did against the goals you set. Then acknowledge all the things you did for yourself, regardless if you fully met your goals or not. Even if your inclination is to zero in on what you didn't complete or how you didn't measure up, stop yourself. Focus first on what you did do and how much you did accomplish. Remember your behavior isn't a reflection of being good or bad, right or wrong. It is a reflection of what you were experiencing at the time you made a choice, and you had reasons for that worth further understanding.

But first pat yourself on the back, give yourself a gold star or just acknowledge that you succeeded in taking better care of yourself the past week. Look at how much you did for yourself and how good that feels – no matter how minimal it may seem.

Then notice if there was anything during or after your aerobic, strengthening or stretching sessions you need to address or get help with. Are you having any stiffness or pain? Are you ready to progress but not sure how to do that? Are you interested in doing something new to add more variety?

Check-ins are also a chance to gain clarity and make different choices. Spend some time looking at the goals you didn't fully make and what you think was really getting in the way. Ask yourself what you can learn from that by seeing it objectively. This isn't a time to be critical but instead to gain insight and understanding about yourself and your situation. And from that clarity, you will get ideas of what will help you succeed. It is always okay to do less, set lower goals or make changes to your routine. The only rules are the ones you decide are best for you.

Weekly Check-In Process

1) Look at what went well and what you did accomplish. This is a time to acknowledge your efforts, give yourself that gold star and periodically reward yourself with something validating – something that isn't food like a new workout item, getting a new outfit or going out for a social event.

2) Check in to how your body is feeling and if you think you need to make any changes to your program or need more professional advice or help.

3) Notice what didn't go as well without any judgment. This helps you be aware of and interested in the choices you made.

4) Also notice if there are patterns in your choices, which could give you more understanding of what is driving your behaviors.

5) Ask yourself if there was anything you would have done differently now that you have 20/20 hindsight. You may not have been able to make different choices. You may have made the best decisions for what was important to you at the time.

6) Now think if there are things you want to change so you can be even more successful next week.

7) Ask yourself some of the coaching questions in this section.

8) And then set new goals for the next week. Be realistic about the type of week you have coming up and set goals you truly believe you can do. If you know you won't have as much time, scale back your goals. If you think you have enough time, consider if you can do a bit more and consider increasing your time or intensity by five percent.

If you decide it helps to check in with someone each week for greater accountability, ask them to withhold any judgment and be there as your sounding board, the one to ask you these questions or as an expert that can give you sound guidance and coaching. Remember you really do have the right answers for yourself.

What reminders or visual cues can you use that will help you remember why you are choosing to be active?

What is motivating to you – is it an end result or seeing what you've done during the week?

Would you be more motivated by seeing how many calories you burned or steps you took?

What do you think will best keep you motivated and on track during the week?

When was the last time you really focused on how your body felt, from your head to your toes?

What will help you pay attention to your limits?

What might get in the way of choosing a reasonable pace you can succeed at?

Where is being fit in your priorities, and is it where you want it to be?

What are ways you can adjust your schedule to make time for exercising or being more active?

Who can support you?

What type of planning and preparation will help you be ready to be active or exercise?

What are you learning from checking in with yourself each week?

Giving Yourself a Chance to Succeed

It may seem obvious you want to set yourself up to succeed, but your past experiences may have you doubting if you really are capable of this. Many of my clients tell me they fear they won't be able to lose weight, stick with the program or really have the success they dream of. This is because they have struggled to follow through in the past. They have a history of not keeping resolutions or maintaining their results after dieting, boot camps, training programs or quick fix supplements. These clients have been disappointed too many times and don't want to set themselves up for failure once more.

If you carry the same beliefs or feelings, you too may be concerned about whether you will fail or be frustrated again. If you aren't sure, start listening to what you are saying to yourself when you think about exercising again or committing to being active more regularly. You may find your self-talk is hard at work to discourage you, warn you of your inadequacies and increase self-doubt.

Negative self-talk is the reason it is important to set yourself up for success every week by choosing things you can do and feel motivated to do and by setting your own pace and goals. You do not have to follow anyone else's rules unless they are designed to fit you, you trust they will serve you, or you have a clear understanding with that person about your limitations, and even then beware if you feel you've been given rules you must adhere to or else. Or else what? Or else you risk being humiliated and lectured to the point you give up? What good is that?

Redefining Success

How you judge if you are a success is tied to your belief system. Most of us believe if we don't meet the full goal, follow the program perfectly or do things exactly as we are told, then we have messed up and been "bad". Where have you heard this in your own life? Are you carrying a belief like this because of something that happened when you were a kid? Perhaps you don't think you were ever good enough or maybe you couldn't please someone no matter what you did right. This is the chance to get clarity through understanding about what is getting in your way of succeeding.

In Doreen's life, she had not been good enough for her father and this was repeated with her husband. In her marriage she did everything she could to please her spouse, but he wasn't impressed and continually put her down, humiliated her in front of others and treated her with disrespect. Doreen tried harder, but nothing she did ever seemed good enough and her attempts at meeting his demands were harshly criticized. She couldn't win, and now she was going through a divorce where he was getting the upper hand. She could see why she was merciless with herself and strived for perfection in everything she did, and she could see what it was costing her.

It is important to be clear on how you are defining success, and how you want to feel when you do succeed. Maybe your definition of success is meeting the prescribed goals no matter what. If so, that is interesting. Or perhaps your definition of success is losing a lot of weight as quickly as possible because if you aren't losing weight you clearly aren't succeeding. It may seem that way, but do you really know if that is true?

Maybe it is time to rethink what it means to succeed with physical fitness. You've been reading that it can feel good to experience the success of being able to do more than you thought, to reach some of your goals even if it isn't all of them and to feel physically better and more confident. Would this feel successful to you?

It is a change in thinking to accept that good is good enough, when you've believed that nothing less than being perfect is acceptable. But consider how freeing it is to do your best on your own terms.

Recognizing Good is Good Enough

This is a good time to rewrite your rules about being a perfectionist and give yourself a break. It is not possible to do everything right all of the time, and for most things it doesn't even matter if you don't come close to doing so. Instead reserve your time and energy to give it your all when it does make a difference, and clearly there are situations in your life for which it matters a great deal.

Whether or not you are active on a given day or for a certain amount of time is seldom that important, unless you are competing, preparing for an event or going through a period when you are deliberately pushing yourself to do more. In the event you choose to work with a personal trainer, which is a good thing to do periodically when you are ready and have the time, you can expect that person to ask more out of you to make some breakthroughs. These are the times when it would matter to strive to do all that you can to meet the requirements.

Otherwise your regular aerobic and fitness goals can accommodate less than perfect compliance. If you have a week (or even a month) when you can't be as active and this occurs during a year when you are active or exercising fairly regularly, you won't even notice or remember that you weren't as active during that time. You would still have results as if you had been active the entire time. This would also be true if every month you had a week when you didn't quite reach your goals. If you find that things come up more often then that, then you need to adjust your goals or look at what is getting in the way.

The idea that you have to be perfect each week is a set up for failure. Instead allow yourself to create a new belief that good is good enough and you will discover that this new thinking will help you succeed for the long-term. When things in your life interfere with your plans, roll with it and see if you can find another time during the week to make it up. If you can't, let it go and keep moving.

If you make a bigger deal out of disruptions and start to beat yourself up, you may determine that you can't succeed and will indeed prove yourself right. You can choose to see things as a minor interruption and let it pass by or you can envision the days you weren't active as a major derailment and struggle to get back on track. It is all in your perspective.

Disruptions are to be expected. Disruptions are not indications of your failure to do as you planned but something to anticipate. Life will often get in the way of your plans. Sometimes it will be for a week and other times for longer periods of time. Instead of letting the missed activity get the best of you or beating yourself up for blowing it, let the judgment and concern go and then get back on track. Sure it will seem more difficult the first time after a week or so of not being active or exercising, but it won't be long before you are back in the swing of things and feeling the motivation return. The important thing is to take that step, even if it is a fraction of what you were doing before — particularly if it's been weeks or months because of a long-term disruption.

What is most important to a fit lifestyle is being consistent, allowing for better weeks than others. With that consistency and increases in your goals you will be doing enough often enough to reach your long-term objectives. If you aren't experiencing any improvement after a few months, then you may need to revisit your goals.

Building a Support Network

It is does take time for both preparation and being active, and this can be difficult without the support from others around you. Many of my clients and show guests have said they couldn't have done it without the support of their families, who agreed to take care of things while they were off doing their fitness routine by juggling their schedules to be home to watch the kids or help with domestic chores. The support they got made all the difference and often facilitated changes in the rest of the family once they could see how much happier, energized and alive the person taking care of themselves became.

It was Elizabeth's husband who gave her the time and money to go to her local gym several nights a week while he took care of the kids. This allowed her to make herself a priority and eliminated her excuse that she couldn't go. She learned not to put herself first and discovered with her husband's support the benefit of taking time out for herself everyday. She's happier, more energized and she feels she is a better wife and mother.

Shann's husband got even more involved, as she shared on the show. Instead of watching TV as they had in the past, he joined her for walks and encouraged her to do other things on her own. When she went through a major derailment period, he noticed the change in her and along with some good friends helped her to find a way to get back on track. He became her partner in creating a healthier lifestyle.

Getting support and having someone there to celebrate your accomplishments along the way are two different things. You might get your family to help you out a bit or maybe your significant other to cover for you, but that doesn't mean they want to hear too much about it. Your friends and colleagues may want to know even less.

Monica's sister and work colleagues were not supportive of her changes as she began working with a trainer and with me as her eating coach. Her colleagues talked behind her back and found ways to sabotage her. Her sister and some of her friends were more obviously hostile to her new behaviors and made things unpleasant. Monica was dismayed by this and realized that she might have to reconsider who her friends were.

As you began to change, your new attitude, lifestyle and appearance may threaten those who aren't doing the same. Their own negative self-judgment, self-talk and hidden beliefs are keeping them from supporting you. More likely they will attempt to sabotage your success with hopes you will stop because they are uncomfortable, and they won't even understand they are doing this to you. This is because they may not be conscious of their behaviors nor understand what is driving them.

It is not uncommon, as you change, to find yourself creating new friends who are aligned to your new interests and activities, whether you have sabotaging people around or not. As Anne and Karen learned, it was natural to develop friends at the gym and in the classes they took. For Anne these new friends became her network because the activities she wanted to do were more about health and they could relate to that. Soon her circle was filled with new friends with healthier interests. This doesn't mean you have to give up old friends, but you may find your social circle will change.

Establishing Accountability

Your support network, as wonderful as it may be, probably isn't the best place to find accountability, and in the first year or so you will likely find you need to be accountable to someone. It is possible to do it for yourself as I did by using the journals and weekly check-ins, but that isn't ideal. I wanted someone to talk to and some support and guidance without hiring a trainer, but I didn't know how to get it.

There are several ways you can now get it. You could ask a good friend or perhaps even your significant other to be your coach and ask you the coaching questions, which will help you in digging a little deeper and gaining more insight. You can turn to one of your new fitness friends who agree with your philosophy and is willing to ask you non-judgmental questions. You can create a group that uses the coaching approach to questions. Or you can hire a professional fitness or wellness coach, who will support you with their own types of questions. More trainers and health experts are getting trained in life and wellness coaching techniques so some may share in this philosophy. And if you want private or group-based healthy lifestyle coaching support that facilitates the concepts in this book with more depth and guidance, you can visit my website.

It is important to find the type of accountability that works for you during the first three to six months — or perhaps even first year — before you have incorporated it fully into your life. People are often amazed that creating healthy changes takes this long, but changing your patterns with fitness and eating is not as simple as creating a new habit in twenty-one days of repetition. There is so much more to changing your lifestyle routines, and for some it takes time to address the underlying emotional and mental mindset issues that are keeping them stuck in old behaviors. How long it takes is irrelevant, what matters is having the support and accountability you need to stick with it until you can't imagine going without your aerobic and fitness activities.

Solving Challenges with Ah-ha Insights & Strategies

Another dimension to success is choosing to learn from your challenges when you don't meet your goals or you feel bored or frustrated to the point you want to give up. As discussed in the preceding section, the weekly check-in process gives you a chance to notice what is getting in the way of doing what you planned to do and being conscious of how you are feeling.

From this neutral perspective, you can start to figure out what you can learn from each week to be even more successful in the future. Those times when you don't make your goals or are struggling in some way are great opportunities to learn more about yourself and to explore new ways of planning, preparing and being active. You can look for the silver lining and make lemonade out of what might initially look like lemons to you. As you look at your patterns or challenges, consider how you might solve them.

One of the problems Maggie had was getting home early enough to get to Curves. Week after week she kept finding she wasn't even coming close to the goals she thought she could make. By the time she got home after a long day and an hour-long commute she was just too exhausted to go out again. She realized that a better solution would be to find a Curves location closer to work, or better yet move closer to work.

Stan on the other hand liked working out in the morning and had a space in the basement where he could do his fitness routine. He enjoyed being active and seeing progress, but he struggled to carve out enough time to see the kind of progress he was looking for. Without judging his choices, he decided to try getting up earlier for one week. That worked. He was soon doubling the amount of time he spent being aerobic and got the results he wanted.

After Ann Marie broke her wrist, she was given a long list of physical therapy exercises she needed to do for the next month to heal properly. She was torn between doing the therapy exercises and finding time for her walks. She just couldn't seem to do both, and she felt badly about it. It was critical she do the wrist exercises, and I suggested she set those as her only goal during that time. If she could get in an occasional walk that would be great, but she needed to focus on healing first. After her wrist healed, she could get back on track with her cardio program. This was the solution she needed to be successful.

Anita loved to walk but not in the heat and humidity of the summer, so she joined a gym as a back-up and found she enjoyed going more than she expected. Soon she became more consistent in her exercising than she thought she could be and was feeling really good about the commitment.

Simone had been in a terrible car accident that required back surgery and had suffered considerable pain ever since. She was afraid to try any type of activity besides walking, for fear it would be too painful or make her symptoms worse. She wanted to do more than just walk and was frustrated. At my encouragement she saw a physical therapist that did a full body evaluation and gave her a series of therapy exercises to do along with recommendations of aerobic activities that wouldn't aggravate her condition. She decided to try them and before long she was successfully and happily using the elliptical trainer and even began using some strengthening equipment. She was so grateful and felt this approach had given her a whole new life.

The issue for Joan was boredom. She loved being active outdoors for long periods of time but during the winter she struggled to spend more than about twenty minutes on her treadmill. We talked about ways to relieve boredom and she came up with the idea of listening to books on tape. She bought a cassette player and began borrowing tapes from the library. This worked and she was excited to tell me, "This is wonderful. It feels like a luxury to have the time to listen to so many books." Soon she was spending forty minutes on the treadmill without a problem as she happily listened to her tapes.

The point is there are all kinds of ways to address whatever is challenging for you. You may not initially see it on your own, but if you ask yourself the coaching questions or talk to a coach advisor you will get a new perspective and ah-ha insights that lead to one or more strategies for resolving the things getting in your way of succeeding.

Coaching Questions to
HAVE A CHANCE TO SUCCEED

What are some of your concerns about your ability to reach your goals and create a healthier lifestyle?

What are you saying to yourself week to week about being more active or meeting your goals?

How are you defining success?

What do you want to feel from being more active?

What beliefs do you have about exercising or getting more fit?

What can you do to get past a derailment or a period when you aren't able to be so active?

Who can help and support you in creating the time for being active and taking care of yourself?

Who can you be accountable to that will withhold judgment and offer a sounding board?

What are you learning doesn't work and what might work better for you?

Progressing and Maintaining Success

When you first start being more active and making it a part of your life, the most exciting aspect is seeing all the changes you make physically, mentally and emotionally. As your body adapts and changes, you will feel you can do even more and will want to amp up your capabilities and try new things to make more improvements. The way to increase activity is through a thoughtful progression, by deliberately increasing the intensity of your routines and by choosing another type or mode of activity to add to your program.

The idea isn't to push yourself too much, but enough that it feels a bit harder to do in a way that feels good. If you push yourself to the point of pain, exhaustion, breathlessness or extreme discomfort it is way too much. The exception is if you are well-conditioned and want to build up anaerobic and aerobic fitness levels by doing cardio interval training mostly above your 85 percent heart rate. At that point I suggest you work with a professional trainer to help you with that type of progression.

To safely progress, the best approach is to listen to your body and when you can easily reach your current goals to increase them by five to ten percent. This works for aerobic or strengthening goals. In addition, mix up your activities and routines and try new things. You will use new muscles and feel more exertion with something different. It is always surprising to me that as fit as I am, I find a new activity more difficult than I would have expected. You probably have had the same experience. By mixing it up, your body can't adapt to what it has become accustomed to and you will get better results.

Increasing Aerobic Progression

If you want to increase your aerobic ability, you can either increase the amount of time, frequency in days or intensity. There becomes a point where the amount of time you can spend is less flexible, so having more options with intensity is what you will use the most.

Aerobic intensity is determined by speed or resistance. Resistance can be going against gravity (as in an incline or hill) or against a weighted resistance (as on a piece of equipment). There is controversy about carrying or wearing weights while being active. While the weights do add resistance, they can also throw off your posture or limit how aerobic you really can become. It is an interesting concept, but I'm inclined to believe you are better off using weights only for strengthening and not when you are focusing on being aerobic.

One of the most powerful ways to enhance your aerobic ability and increase your results is the use of interval training. You've probably seen interval programs on cardio equipment. By increasing and decreasing your exertion as you move, you are forcing your body to work harder while giving it a chance to recover and avoid exceeding 85 percent of your maximum heart rate for any length of time. It is fine when you have been consistently doing moderately hard levels to use intervals that exceed the aerobic threshold in controlled short periods that allows for enough recovery back under 85 percent, but don't try this if you haven't acclimated yourself to RPE levels of 6-8.

There are many ways to create an interval program, and you will frequently see interval recommendations in fitness magazines. Generally they are designed to work you up to a high level, let you recover, and then repeat that a number of times. The rule of thumb is twice or three times the recovery period for however long you pushed yourself. So if you exert yourself for thirty seconds, slow down for one or two minutes. If you push hard for one minute, give yourself two or three minutes to recover at a slower pace before doing another set. When you are much more aerobically fit, you can experiment with less recovery and more time spent in the anaerobic zone to further increase your aerobic fitness.

A great way to really get in touch with your body, monitor your actual level of intensity and do interval routines is with a heart rate monitor (with a chest band transmitter and watch). For many of my clients, a heart rate monitor is also quite motivating and fun to use. It can also make your activity time more interesting as you use the monitor to determine when to increase and decrease your exertion levels.

You can get a heart rate monitor almost anywhere, but many have limited features or force you to set up the watch using the standard 220 minus your age formula. I've learned that while many people do fit the formula, just as many don't. In addition, not all monitors are accurate or reliable. Many of my colleagues and I prefer the Polar brand. But I'll warn you in advance that even these higher-end monitors have quirks and will have times when they don't show a reading, will spike a reading too high or seem not to work properly. It can be frustrating. You might want to do your own research to see what brands and features are best for you.

Sarah did start using the heart rate monitor and really enjoyed it. She liked knowing her zones and controlling her heart rate as she did her activities. She played around with different interval programs and would wear her monitor when she did new activities to see how much exertion they required. She came to have a pretty good idea of what it would say based on her rate of perceived exertion and she liked the confidence of knowing how her body was doing and how it was feeling to make better decisions.

DAY	DATE		Type of Activity	Minutes	Intensity / Heart Rate Avg	Calories Burned	Steps Taken	Stretches	Yoga
		GOAL	Walk	50	4-6				
		ACTUAL	Walk	50	125	392		5	3
M	4-10	COMMENT	I got a good pace going and added some intervals that felt really good						
		GOAL							
		ACTUAL							3
T	4-11	COMMENT							
		GOAL	Richard Simmons	40	6-8				
		ACTUAL	Richard Simmons	40	137	401		5	3
W	4-12	COMMENT							
		GOAL							
		ACTUAL							
TH	4-13	COMMENT							
		GOAL	Aerobic class	60	6-8				
		ACTUAL							
F	4-14	COMMENT	Didn't make it tonight but I'll try for it again next week						
		GOAL							
		ACTUAL	Walk	65	129	292		5	3
S	4-15	COMMENT	Great walk today. The weather was amazing and it was great to get out and enjoy it. I had one hill for the interval.						
		GOAL	Leslie Sansone	45	5-8				
		ACTUAL	Leslie Sansone	45	141	427		3	3
S	4-16	COMMENT	This was a bit tough but I kept my heart rate under 150 most of the time, so it was okay						
		TOTALS		200		1512			

Strengthening Progression

If you want to increase your strength, you could increase the resistance (as in the weight or thickness of tubing) as well as the number of sets. The basic guidelines for strengthening are as follows:

	Frequency**	Sets	Repetitions	Exercises
Beginner	2 times/week	1 set	10-15 reps*	Whole body
Endurance	2 times/week	2-3 sets	12-15 reps	Whole body
Strength	3-4 times/wk	3 sets	8-12 reps	Upper and lower body

* Repetitions are the number of times a specific exercise is performed in a set
** Frequency: Muscles need at least 48 hours (2 days) of recovery. After 4 days the muscle begins to lose what it gained, which is why the frequency recommendation is at least 2 times a week.

The objective is for the resistance to be enough that you can do the minimum number of repetitions before you fatigue at or before reaching the maximum number. For example, you might be doing a bicep curl with ten pound weights. It will be the right weight for you if you can complete at least eight of them but not more than twelve or fifteen repetitions. You will know you are fatigued when you can no longer perform the exercise properly and are using other parts of your body to try to complete the repetition.

In the past, there was one primary approach to strengthening and now many more ways to do strengthening exercises are available. You can do strength training that isolates one muscle using equipment, tubing or free weights and using the guidelines for strengthening (see the 3rd line in the chart above). Or you could do something called functional training that uses the endurance guidelines (the 2nd line) with lesser weight and often combines two exercise movements at a time while you are standing or even balancing on something. You will see routines for both of these types in many of the fitness magazines.

Isometric exercises also work, in which you use your muscle in a static position to resist against gravity or some other type of force for ten or fifteen seconds. Isometric exercises are often included in video programs or yoga classes. Variations on other types of strengthening are also being added to Pilates, yoga, videos and fitness classes.

Before you start doing strengthening, learn how to do the exercises properly. I highly recommend you work with a trainer for a while to understand how to hold your body, perform the routine properly and become familiar with progression. You may want to meet with a trainer twice a week for at least a month to be sure you fully understand what you are doing and can perform the routine correctly on your own.

If you have ever had physical therapy, I encourage you to pull out those old exercises and start doing them in advance of starting a strengthening program. Very often old injuries can create chronic muscle imbalances that you don't notice and that can lead to re-injury once you start being more active. I also encourage you to see a physical therapist if you are over forty or have any aches or pains that are bothering you before you start strengthening. As we age, our posture and daily activities can lead to muscle imbalances that sets you up to be an injury waiting to happen, just as I once was. Many people pull muscles and hurt themselves while strength training and this can be minimized with physical therapy preparation.

Staying Motivated to Maintain New Behaviors

Once you have been active and progressively increasing your abilities, you might think you will get to a point where you don't need to worry about staying motivated. To a certain degree that is true. After a year or so, and everyone is different as to when this happens, you no longer fight the process and will miss how it feels when you can't be active. But you may still have times when you lose interest or get derailed and have to get back on track. This is why it helps to do things you love and look forward to as you build activity into your lifestyle.

This becomes even more important when you reach the goals you set out in your initial vision, and you shift into maintenance. At this point you won't see the kind of results that occurred in the first year or two and instead you will plateau for longer periods of time. Yet this is also a great opportunity to explore new things and expand your fitness goals because you will be fit, confident and interested to see what else you can do.

People of all ages are participating in greater numbers in races, triathlons, biking events, active vacations and hiking clubs. You are not limited, and having met your initial goals you know what your body can do and what might interest you. This is a great time to sign up for things you've never tried and take your fitness to new heights of capability or add a different modality completely, like Tai Chi.

I have discovered that I want to add something new every year, and I have an array of things that I can and like to do each week. I started off with my StairMaster that first year and added strength training using traditional free weight exercises the second year. In my third year I started practicing Pilates and then added rowing my fourth. The fifth year I started kickboxing instruction and learned how to do functional strengthening, and last year I added in some yoga and skip roping. I still do a mix of all these things regularly. This year I'm interested in dancing and trying a rock climbing wall. Rock climbing would have been the last thing I would have considered back when I started. Now it sounds like fun.

Your perspective shifts the more active you are. I have learned the more I do, the more I can and want to do. Whereas the less I do, the less I can or will have an interest in doing. The beauty of feeling good from physical movement is that you don't have to force yourself to do more. It will happen on its own. You will find ways to stay motivated to maintain your new behaviors because you have stayed active long enough to get to this point and it just feels too good to stop.

Creating a New Motivating Vision

Once you have reached your vision for why you wanted to become more active and fit in the first place, you may want to consider creating a new vision. Maybe you can now see yourself in a triathlon in another year or biking across Europe. If so you have some planning and goal setting to do. If you don't consider the possibility of what else you want to achieve, you might not attempt it. On the other hand, not everyone is motivated by long-term visions once they get to this point and just want to keep living an active lifestyle. You know what works for you.

Now is a good time to write down what you've accomplished, how it makes you feel and what has worked to keep you on track. Some day you may have a significant derailment and you will be glad you have this to help you find your way back to where you are now.

Recognizing and Celebrating How Good You Feel

It is a wonderful feeling to know you have succeeded in embracing an active lifestyle and reached your goals, whether it was week-to-week or the goals you set out at the onset. You will value how you feel about yourself and your body, and it won't be based on what you weigh or the size of your clothes – not that you won't notice these, but you won't care the way you would have expected.

Celebrating Your Successes

It is important to celebrate your success and acknowledge what you've accomplished, and hopefully you've been doing that all along the way. Consider what would be a way of celebrating your success that rewards you for sticking with your changes. Would it be rewarding to go somewhere special, take a trip, wear something new, buy a piece of fitness equipment, join a class or pamper yourself in some way? Pick something on a regular basis to help you acknowledge and value your achievements.

Giving Yourself Time to Adjust to the New You

It also helps to recognize that a part of you may not fully acknowledge your changes. You may not recognize yourself in the mirror for a couple of years and instead see the old image of yourself. When I lost a lot of weight many years ago from dieting, I kept being surprised by how slim my legs were. They didn't look like my legs, and it was years before I accepted them as my own. More recently it took me time to really believe how solid and toned my legs were and that I no longer had cellulite practically down to my knees. I kept looking for signs of it for at least a year after it was gone. I hear stories from many other people who have gone through similar experiences. You can take the fat out the girl or boy, but it takes longer to take the fat girl or boy out of who they become.

Give yourself time to adjust to the new you and with getting attention for your new body and attitude. For some people this is unwanted attention and perhaps the very reason they were out of shape and overweight in the first place. Yet in the process of changing your body, you will also changing your beliefs and self-esteem, and you will be better prepared to deal with the increased attention. The best thing to do is thank people when they compliment you and allow yourself to receive how good it feels to be recognized for your accomplishments. You do deserve it after all.

Coaching Questions to
CELEBRATE HOW GOOD YOU FEEL

What would be a way you can celebrate your successes that feels empowering and validating?

How can you remind yourself to recognize your accomplishments?

What about your new appearance is hardest to accept and how could you start to acknowledge it with grace and love for yourself?

Being Satisfied with
Healthier Eating

Nearly everyone likes the idea of eating in a healthier way and has tried various diets to do just that. Yet dieting isn't the same thing as healthy eating. In fact, it often leads to unhealthy and dysfunctional eating.

Sadly, many people no longer know or feel confident about how to make healthy food choices. The struggle to eat well has primarily occurred because of the emphasis on weight loss and looking for the illusive answer to getting thin. The many different types of diets, constantly changing research findings and rotating publicized experts has taken something that is actually very simple and complicated it. As we can all see, those experts and diets haven't led to an answer that everyone can succeed with. That means you and many others are still looking for something that actually does work.

You may think you know what diet is supposed to work. People often tell me they know what to eat; they just can't seem to do it as often as they know they should. My experience tells me that very few people have a good handle on what foods are actually healthy, how to shop for healthier foods or easy ways to prepare meals. They have heard or tried so many different recommendations and come to their own conclusions, that the end result is both unhealthy and unsatisfying. Being dissatisfied with food choices (and then with oneself in many cases) is one of the main reasons people overeat or choose things that aren't that healthy.

Your experience with food is meant to be satisfying, and what I will show you in this section is how to eat in a healthier way that is enjoyable, allows for all foods in moderation, fits into your life and frees you of the guilt. I won't tell you what you can or can't eat. Instead I will free you to eat what you discover makes you feel your best and what you enjoy eating most. The most amazing experience happens when you give yourself permission to enjoy your food while paying attention to how you feel physically. You will find you want less of the junk and more of what is healthier, and it isn't an internal battle that requires willpower. Eating for physical and emotional satisfaction is something you genuinely want to do.

The challenge is overcoming the diet mindset that has been an integral part of our culture. Diets do not work for ninety-five percent of those that do them, and there is more evidence of this everyday. In the past twenty years obesity has dramatically increased. Those twenty years (from 1986 to 2006) coincide with the low-fat dieting that started in the mid 1980s and low-carbohydrate diets that followed in the late 1990s. Women, on average, have tried ten diets during their lives, and these include Weight Watchers and low-carb diets. Men in contrast only started dieting in high numbers about fifteen years ago as they became more conscious of their appearance, and most of them have also experimented with the low-carb diets. If you'll notice, more men are struggling with their weight today than in the past, and it isn't just the beer belly anymore.

Statistics from the U.S. Centers for Disease Control show us that two thirds of the population is now overweight and a third of these are obese. Nearly a third of American children are also obese. Obesity more than doubled between 1980 (then at fifteen percent) and 2004 (to become thirty-three percent). And these numbers have continued to go up every year.

Yet these are not just numbers. These are real people. They are us and the people we know and love. They represent the painful reality of what dieting has done to our culture and to ourselves. Not only do most people believe diets are the only way to get thin and reach the ideal, they believe that if they don't succeed at sticking with them, or worse regain the weight, that they have failed, don't have enough willpower or are out of control. The more often this happens, the less confident these people feel about themselves, the more they weigh, and the lower their self-esteem becomes. The impact of how people feel about themselves from dieting often shows up in other parts of their lives.

Carolyn is a good example. She always focused on how bad she'd been during the week when checking in with me. She was quick to point out she was bad when she ate too many cookies on one day and couldn't stop overeating at night on another. She also believed she was bad because she didn't meet all her fitness goals, and she would beat herself up for not taking better care of herself. Where did she get the idea she was so bad all the time? As we began to remove the belief she was bad with food in our sessions, I noticed the word "bad" was disappearing from her vocabulary even in reference to other aspects of her life. I see this change a lot with other clients too, and when it happens I know they are on their way to reclaiming their power and freedom with more than just food.

Diets promise quick weight loss and being in control. While the promise appears to be fulfilled when on the diet, inevitably you succumb to forbidden foods, struggle to stick with the plan, or stop doing the diet when you reach your goal weight. When that happens the see saw (and for some the roller coaster) begins. With few exceptions, the first thing people do after a diet is eat and drink to their heart's content the things that were restricted on the diet. Many gorge on these forbidden foods and beverages, making up for what they missed out on and enjoying the reward of their accomplishment.

But at the same time, hidden below the surface, is a voice that reminds you that what you are doing is bad and you really shouldn't be doing it. This voice is tied to your belief system that bought into the diet rules, and it will monitor your choices and criticize you for making bad decisions. Another part of you doesn't want to be told what to do and will compensate for the criticism by overeating or choosing the "bad foods" anyway. The associated guilt and feeling you are indeed bad for your behavior only creates more of this dynamic. The see saw is the internal struggle to be good one day, only to be bad the next, and the battle to stay in control. For many this transitions into a roller coaster of perpetual on-again-off-again dieting and bingeing.

The way off the see saw and roller coaster is to first become aware you are on it by becoming conscious of your behaviors and what you are telling yourself, and then to address the beliefs and feelings that keep you stuck. This consciousness raising and positive-change process is based on the 3 Cs.

Applying the 3 Cs to Healthier Eating

As a society, we've been conditioned since children to eat when and what we are told and then to eat everything on our plates. Unfortunately these well-meaning household rules disengage us from being connected to our hunger levels, desire for nutritious foods and intuitive sense of satisfaction.

We are taught to eat according to a household schedule and the beliefs of those feeding us. For some people, that means eating at specific times whether they are hungry or not. For many others, it means eating everything on the plate no matter how full they've become. And for younger generations, it means skipping meals and grabbing food on the run. Any rules governing your eating behaviors, whether it was to get you to eat less or more of something or do it a specific way, adds to the disconnection with your own instincts about what, when and how much to eat.

As a result, you probably determine how much to eat and pick your foods subconsciously, and you don't know what it really feels like to be hungry, satisfied or full. You probably don't know if you really like the foods you are eating or what drives you to eat the way you do. Regaining awareness and making choices based on your understanding of how you feel physically, mentally, emotionally and even spiritually is the key to being in control.

Consciousness without Judgment

As I discussed in part 2, awareness of your behaviors and choices is what makes it possible to change them. Becoming a neutral and curious observer instead of a judgmental critic provides a safe way to gain insight about what drives your actions.

You can start raising your consciousness by looking at what has driven you to diet in the past and to what extent you still want to diet. By getting in touch with the beliefs or feelings that has put you on the see saw of restricting and overeating, you can understand what it is that you need or want for yourself.

Dieting, for my client Janice, was a way of feeling in control and hopeful about her future. It wasn't so much that she wanted to diet, it was the belief that it was the only thing that would work and it was something that others around her would support. Yet she knew, deep down, diets didn't work for her and she wanted a more sane way of eating that felt better and could be integrated into her life. She hated how she felt when she blew the diet or went out of control when off the diet. She was sick of the whole thing and was ready for a new way of approaching food that was healthy and reinforcing.

Many others I've worked with dieted primarily to lose weight and didn't feel good about themselves unless they were a certain weight. They struggled to see they were amazing for who they were, regardless of their size. Some couldn't find two things they liked about themselves. Unfortunately losing weight doesn't change how you feel about yourself, and sadly many people are disappointed with themselves even at a size 8, 4 or 2. For them the problem isn't their weight as much as their self-worth. Once they are conscious of this disconnect, they begin to focus on what really matters and address ways to enhance their self-confidence, health and happiness.

The way to eating healthier relies on being conscious of how you feel physically and emotionally and observing what you are doing and thinking when you are around food. As you will discover in this section, that isn't as tough to do as you might imagine. The first step is being conscious of when you get hungry, satisfied and full by using the hunger scale and discovery journal that I'll describe in Getting Started Consciously on page 136. Greater consciousness will happen quite easily and you'll find yourself becoming more aware of your hunger levels without much effort at all. In fact many of my clients are surprised how fast they start becoming conscious and how naturally it occurs.

Clarity through Understanding

As you become more conscious, you will start to notice how often you are hungry but don't eat, eat beyond the point of being satisfied or eat when you aren't even hungry.

Once you have the awareness, you can then begin to investigate what is behind those actions. Dieting and the way you were raised has conditioned you not to notice when you are even doing these things, as Brandy was surprised to find out when she overate on a regular basis. Once you do notice the patterns you can begin to identify what is causing you to eat the way you do.

There are many reasons you might overeat, as you learned in part 2. It could be because you haven't had enough food all day, have primarily eaten just carbohydrates, are mindlessly eating, have associated food with the situation you are in, are feeling pressured to eat, are being driven by subconscious beliefs, have been denied what you want, or you are repressing feelings and turning to food to cope.

It doesn't help to make an assumption before you further investigate what is really going on, as I often remind my clients. You may be convinced your issue is emotional eating, sugar addiction, laziness, or lack of motivation, but that may not turn out to be the case. Instead you may discover that it is something very different and easily explainable and resolvable.

The process of self-discovery allows you to see what is driving your decisions, causing you to over or under eat. With each insight, you will be able to gain greater clarity, try new things, alter your beliefs and experiment with tactics to see what helps you eat in a way that is more wholesome, balanced and fulfilling. By compassionately understanding yourself better, you will overcome the diet mindset and beliefs that don't serve you and instead create ways of integrating healthier eating behaviors into your life on your own terms.

Choices without Deprivation or Need for Perfection

These terms include choices that you feel free to make even if others think you shouldn't. If you are told you can't have something, particularly a favorite food, you will think more about it and likely want it to the point of obsession. It is human nature to want what we can't have and this is why dieting generally leads to overeating and bingeing.

When you have been deprived, anticipate being deprived or believe you should be deprived, you have set the stage for a battle between your internal enforcing parent and willful child who has needs. The louder, more demanding and critical the enforcer becomes, the more the deprived child acts up and rebels against the rigid parental controls. This scenario also tends to replay dynamics from your past that represent unresolved experiences and unmet needs that are typically loaded with unexpressed emotions.

The way to deal with the inner enforcer trying to get you to do what you should and the child determined to get what it wants is to calm them both down by giving each a little of what they need. This may seem counter intuitive, as it once did to me. You might think it is better to change your beliefs and disregard the enforcing voice, and to some extent that works. But I've learned that the parental enforcer and reactive child are parts of our persona and not something you can remove. Instead they serve a useful purpose in helping us understand our beliefs and emotions.

The enforcer (or whatever name you come up for it) has the job of enforcing what you believe to be true. If you believe you can't have certain foods, are bad if you do or remember being told not to have specific foods growing up, your enforcer is working hard to keep you in line. If you believe you must be perfect to be good or loved, your enforcer reminds you that nothing less than perfection is acceptable. If you deviate, the inner critic (another one of your voices) won't mince words and will mimic the worst things that have ever been said to you or blow them out of proportion. Start to pay attention to what your voices are saying to you, and you will get insight into your beliefs and where they are coming from.

The deprived child (or the free spirit as one client calls it) has the job of helping you get your emotional needs met. Maybe you were denied your favorite foods as a child or told you were fat and needed to diet. You are carrying emotions from those experiences. Perhaps you are feeling unworthy, empty or unlovable from a past or current situation and want some comfort. Or maybe you are upset, stressed or frustrated and need something to help you get through the day. These are all real and valid feelings and needs. So too is the desire to eat foods you enjoy and taste yummy, no matter what the enforcer says. If you watch the way you are reacting, you can get in touch with your needs and desires that aren't being met.

Acknowledging and validating these parts of yourself helps you to see the struggle. The way to calm the voices down involves changing your beliefs about good and bad foods, when and how much you should eat, and the need for perfection in following your diet. Notice this removes dichotomous thinking of all or nothing and right or wrong. When you choose to allow all foods in moderation, there is less rigidity or territorial boundaries. When you eat according to your body's hunger signals and balance your foods, there is more emphasis on what feels healthy, enjoyable and satisfying. These two techniques are reassuring to the enforcer, who no longer needs to police your choices, and the child who doesn't need to overreact to be soothed. I will be explaining more about how to work with these voices further on in this section.

The hardest part of this process is changing your beliefs about certain foods. Depending on the number of diets you've been on or the research you've taken to heart, your list of perceived bad foods may be extensive. You may have, as one of my clients did, a very short list of what you think you should eat. Her fear was that I was going to shorten it even further, and she wasn't sure how she would handle it. Instead I helped her to see that the list could be expanded. Much like the box people get in with exercise where the only place they believe they can go to get fit is the gym, another box gets created around being good with food where the only answer is dietary restrictions, a limited list of acceptable foods and complete compliance.

When you have the option to choose what you love in a way that is healthy and unrestricted, you experience the pleasure of eating without guilt. It is a great feeling to be free of the baggage and the box you once felt you couldn't get yourself out of.

Finding Your Motivation

Any significant change in your lifestyle requires enough motivation to adopt new behaviors and stick with them for the long term. As I discussed in Being Active, it is usually a defining moment that leads you to take action and a vision of what you want in your life to help you stick with your new routines.

For most people being overweight becomes the catalyst in changing the way they eat. Sarah is a good example. She called me because she was having trouble losing weight and had done several diets to no avail. In fact she said she was only getting heavier. I've already discussed several reasons why focusing on your weight sabotages your efforts, and I'll add one more. The more you focus on something, the more you give it substance in your reality.

This is aligned with the *Laws of Attraction* that states what you focus on with your thoughts and emotions becomes your reality. So if you are focused on being overweight or too fat, you are giving energy to that reality. Eva Gregory, a master Law of Attraction coach and author of *The Feel Good Guide to Prosperity*, once said "The reason diets don't work is you go on a diet to get rid of the fat you don't want. So where is your focus? On the fat! So what are you attracting more of? Fat! Exactly what you don't want!" This kind of thinking will put you back in the diet mindset, and that will make it nearly impossible to free yourself from past beliefs, emotions or behaviors.

Coming to Terms with the Diet Mindset

This is a good time to come to grips with how you feel and what you believe about diets. There is a lot about dieting that is no doubt familiar and perhaps even comforting to you. You may like the structure, camaraderie, initial proof something is working or even the specific shopping lists and recipes. This is important to know about yourself, so you can either understand why these things matter and then let them go or incorporate them into your new routines.

You may also like the way diets make you feel in control or supported as Janice did. If that's the case, what other feelings or beliefs are behind these for you? Do you carry a belief that without the enforcer you can't be good and will fail? If so, isn't that interesting and where does that come from? If you can be in control and succeed elsewhere in your life, you have evidence that you can handle yourself around food as well. That recognition that you can be in control will support you in changing your beliefs.

Perhaps you feel judged by others for what you eat or those around you have said you should be on a diet. That is their judgment and just because they believe this doesn't make it right or true. You can choose to be the victim of their judgment or stand up for what is best for your health and self-esteem.

And last but not least, you may believe dieting is the primary and best way to lose weight, particularly if you've had some success before. While it is easy to believe this and the dieting industry has worked hard to convince us of it, it isn't true. The way to successfully lose weight and keep it off is to raise your metabolism, and the only way to do that is by increasing your activity level and muscle while fueling this higher demand for energy with more nutritious calories – not less. Restricting food reduces your metabolism. If you restrict your calories often enough, you will lower your metabolism to the point that it becomes fairly difficult to raise in the future.

You may be in this situation now, if you've done many diets, have stopped seeing the kind of results you once got when you first started dieting, or you are close to or at your heaviest weight. This means, that like me, it will take time to see any weight loss as you begin to heal your body and work to raise your metabolism. It takes patience to both fix and increase your metabolic rate, which is what will give you long-term weight loss success. In the meantime, the best thing is to focus on the other benefits that come from eating healthier, such as feeling better and having more energy.

Identifying What Really Motivates You

The real question is why it is important to you to eat in a healthier way. What is motivating you to change the way you eat? Sure weight loss may be part of that, but what will that give you? How will that make you feel? What is it about being overweight or unhealthy that isn't allowing you to have or experience what you want in your life?

FIND YOUR MOTIVATION

Catalyst Motivators

When have you recently experienced angst about your weight, health or fitness?

What was upsetting about these situations?

Were you motivated by any of these to make a change?

What steps did you take to address your eating habits?

How long did you stay motivated to continue with your new behaviors?

What do you believe was the greatest challenge in staying on track?

To what extent do you think the diet mentality sabotaged your ability to succeed?

Feel Good Motivators

Why is it important to you to lose weight, be fit or get healthier?

What will you be able to experience or do in your life that you can't do now?

What is that you want to feel?

When in your life did you feel that way before, and how can you see yourself regaining this feeling?

On a scale of 0 – 10, how motivated are you to start eating healthier as a lifestyle? (0 being not motivated, 10 being highly motivated)

If you are under a 7, what can you do to feel more motivated?

Getting Started Consciously

Just the thought of getting started may be driving you to grab more food and go on a binge fest. While you may understand this isn't going to be a diet, part of you probably doesn't believe it. You may even decide you aren't ready for this yet and may come back to this section several times before deciding to give it a try.

It is normal to feel some anxiety about starting yet another program designed to change the way you eat. So let me reassure you now that this process will not restrict the foods you love to eat or force you to radically change your behaviors in a way that is unpleasant. Instead you will learn how you can have your cake, really enjoy it and then feel good about eating it. "No guilt, no grief," as Heather Moreno says in her book *Achieving Physical Wealth*, where she challenges the rules of eating and exercise to achieve better results.

The approach I'm about to share with you is very different from being given a dietary plan of specific foods you can eat, calories you must meet per day, a journal to ensure you follow the guidelines, and weekly weigh-ins to measure results. The benefit of a specific dietary plan and compliance program is you don't have to think for yourself and you can just follow the rules. The disadvantage is the preoccupation with food, weight and thoughts about whether you are being good or bad, which keeps you stuck in the diet mentality.

A better way to be in control and change your relationship with food is to take the focus off of food, calorie counting and weight. Have you ever heard or read the statement, "It isn't about the food?" It is true. The struggle to eat in a healthy way is seldom about the food or the beverage; it is much deeper than that. So unlike any other book you've read about eating healthier or program you have tried, I am not going to start off focusing on food or what you should eat.

Instead, we will focus on how you feel when you eat physically, mentally and emotionally, and by doing this you will get to know which foods don't feel that good to you and why you wanted them in the first place. While this isn't as simple as following a dietary plan at first, it is actually easier and becomes an enjoyable process as you get more in touch with yourself. Once you really feel the impact of what and why you eat, you will choose to eat differently and won't want to go back to diets or unhealthy choices.

You may appreciate this as Maggie did when she wrote me and said, "Thank you for not making me just stop drinking Pepsi and eat less, which is the message I have been hearing from all the places I have turned the past few years." She drank large quantities of Pepsi throughout the day, and she feared she had a sugar addiction that no one, not even Overeaters Anonymous, had been able to help her resolve. I told her right up front that the last thing I would do is tell her to stop having Pepsi. Instead I would give her a way of having permission that would put her in charge of her choices with the Pepsi.

Imagine how relieved Maggie (and her inner child) felt, knowing the Pepsi wouldn't be taken away. It is much easier to start a new behavior knowing it won't be drastic or upsetting. You can relax into it and be open to exploring what is driving unhealthy choices without fear of reprisals. Within a month of starting the process Maggie no longer felt she had an addiction and two months later she was drinking Pepsi once in a while. It had been easy to drink less of it, and she had made all her own choices about if or when she had a Pepsi. She never once felt forced to change her behaviors, instead she gravitated to the changes from within herself. The problem wasn't an addiction; it was an outlet for subconscious emotions and beliefs. Once she understood that she knew what to do and the change was painless.

The challenge in explaining my process is that you are very different from everyone else in what you believe, feel and struggle with regarding food and possibly beverages. No two people have the same issues or mindset because everyone's past environments and experiences are totally different.

Unlike helping people get active, which is more sequential, this is more of a zigzag process and driven by what is getting in your way of making healthier choices. As a result, you may find that some of the information in this section either doesn't apply to you or that the sections on Making Healthier Choices and Addressing Emotional Hunger should be in reverse order. I recommend you read through it all first before getting started, and then you can decide whether dealing with your food choices or your mindset need to come first for you.

Recognizing Physical Hunger Signals

Regardless of the order you choose to follow in this section, the one practice that does come first is getting in touch with how your body feels physically. You've been taught a lot about how to eat during your life, but you haven't been taught how to be conscious of your hunger signals or how to know the difference between physical, mental or emotional hunger so you can respond accordingly to your needs.

Our hunger signals tell us when we are hungry, satisfied or full, and provide a natural mechanism for portion control. Each of us feels these signals a bit differently. For me, I get an unpleasant gnawing sensation that feels warm when I get hungry and cold, irritable and slightly nauseous if I get too hungry. When I'm full I feel bloated, heavy and have an ache in my stomach. I know I am satisfied when I feel fulfilled, content and don't have any desire for more food, which is more of an intuitive knowing that I've had enough. For you the signals could be quite different.

You may be vaguely aware of your hunger signals, or as many of my clients discover, you may not really know what it really feels like to be hungry, satisfied or full.

To help you start to get in touch with your levels of hunger, the best tool to use is the hunger scale. It is a simple gauge that runs from 0 to 10.

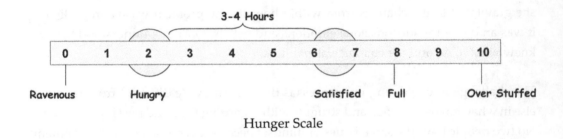

Hunger Scale

At 0 you are ravenous and often past the point of feeling any hunger, and at 10 – at the other extreme – you are sickeningly stuffed. In between going up the scale from 0, you are very hungry at 1, hungry at 2, getting an early signal of getting hungry at 3, and not much of anything until you reach a 6 or 7. Between a 6 and 7 you are satisfied after having eaten, which is the feeling of having enjoyed your food, being satiated and not needing anything more. There is seldom a physical sensation to this. It is more contentment and a knowing that what you had was just right. When you reach 8 you are full, and 9 is uncomfortably full.

When you are hungry at a 2, your body is letting you know that metabolically you need fuel and your blood sugar levels are likely falling. When you get to an 8 and start feeling full, you are getting too much fuel for what your body needs and the excess will be stored as fat and your blood sugars are probably getting too high.

If you eat when you are hungry (2) and stop before getting full between a 6 and 7, you will find yourself getting hungry every three to four hours and eating about five times during the day. The beauty of this is you will be continually fueling your metabolism and keeping your blood sugars from going too low or too high, particularly if you eat foods that are a balance of protein, carbohydrates and fat. I will cover balanced eating later in this section since I don't want you to get too focused on that just yet. In the meantime, when I use the term balance it is in reference to balancing foods so they include a mix of healthy carbohydrates, proteins and fats in a meal or snack.

For now, it is more important to focus on your hunger level sensations and really understand what they feel like for you and to notice them. Unfortunately dieting has taught us to deny our hunger and to find ways to avoid eating for as long as possible. As a result, many people don't often feel hungry or are pleased when they can let the hunger feeling pass, believing they are no longer hungry. This only sets them up for overeating when they finally do eat and further depressing their metabolism.

The way Simone helped herself pay attention to her hunger levels was to set an alarm on her computer about three hours after she last ate so she could stop and check in with herself, otherwise she would work right through her hunger during the day and never notice it. Setting alarms in your calendar (like Microsoft's Outlook program) works really well and many of my clients have done it to help them gain awareness of their hunger, particularly midmorning and midday. They are often surprised that the hunger signal is there when they stop to notice, and the more they are aware of it the stronger it becomes, eliminating the need to use the alarm to gain their attention.

Diane was amazed when she started paying attention to hunger levels. "No diet had ever given me a way to listen to my body, and I'm aware of it for the first time." By the second week she realized she wasn't eating enough during the day and in the third week of being conscious of her hunger she began eating breakfast and feeling much better. Jill was worried she wouldn't know if she was hungry or full because she didn't think she had ever felt this before. But within a week or so she was starting to feel both types of signals and after a few weeks began to really isolate the different types of sensations along the scale.

Some people find it easier than others to identify the different sensations. It took Brandy five days to become fully aware of her hunger levels, and she disliked the feeling of being full so much she immediately stopped overeating. For Daphne it took a few weeks to figure out the levels around being hungry and full. When she did distinguish them, she realized she was eating at a 3 and not waiting long enough to be hungry. She also began to really feel fullness and was able to see ways she could cut back. The process of being conscious was quite profound for her because it exemplified her rushed lifestyle and how little attention she was paying to herself.

Many others find it takes longer to fully recognize each of the stages of the scale and to be conscious of it on a daily basis. The most exciting breakthrough for them and for me is when they start feeling hungry more often. It is a eureka moment because it means their metabolism is more engaged and they are shifting out of their old patterns and beliefs that enabled hunger denial.

My client Maria knew she skipped too many meals, but her travel schedule and work life demands didn't leave much room for stopping to eat. The more conscious she became of how she felt, the more respectful she became of the signals. After six weeks she began to see how hungry she really was and after twelve weeks she was listening so well she ate every three to five hours, in keeping with her body's need to refuel. She was honoring her hunger and respecting her fullness, and in the process honoring and respecting herself, and she liked how that felt.

Annette found that she routinely waited to eat until she was ravenous, at the point she didn't feel anything at all. Be aware that when you stop feeling hungry DOES NOT mean you are no longer hungry. You are. Your body just doesn't let you feel the pain associated with that, which is how we survived long periods without food years ago.

Annette also frequently skipped breakfast and drank lots of water instead. She resisted breakfast because she had been convinced as a teenager that to lose weight the best thing was to just have water in the morning. It had clearly never worked. She had been dealing with weight issues her entire adult life, but she still subconsciously held on to that belief. We also discovered she stopped eating at about a level 5, not wanting to eat too much. As a result, she never quite met her body's demand for food and found herself snacking frequently during the day and feeling out of control. Much like Maria, she began to really notice her hunger after six weeks and was responding to her hunger signals and eating at a 2 and stopping closer to a 7 regularly by the twelfth week. She was then eating enough food to satisfy and energize herself.

Stuart found the process of experimenting and paying attention to his levels fun. He was able to observe how his body felt and to become familiar with the times he was more prone to overeat. Once he knew his hunger level signals he found it was easy to recognize satisfaction and stop before getting full, and this gave him a feeling of confidence with food and portion control.

We are blessed to have an innate signaling system to help us eat normally, which you can see at work with young children. They know when they are hungry and ask for food, and they know when they are satisfied and done before getting full. It is intuitive to them, and the good news is we can reclaim that ability ourselves by being in touch with our sensations and intuition on a regularly basis.

Understanding Satisfaction

Identifying when satisfaction occurs is more difficult because it is an intuitive feeling rather than a physical one. There is no feeling of hunger or fullness when you are eating, so you don't have any sensation to guide you. Instead you are relying on a feeling of being satisfied and satiated without becoming full, which is more an experience of pleasure and a knowing that you are all set and don't need anything more to become satisfied.

If you tend to often eat to the point of being full at an 8, try having a few less bites than you normally eat and see where a 7 is on the scale for you. If you want to aim for a 6, try having about a fourth less and see if you can still be satisfied with that. Soon you will simply know where you are on the scale. You will know when you are done and fulfilled, or you will know you need a bit more to be satisfied.

Surprisingly, most of us aren't encouraged to be satisfied when we eat. We aren't taught to savor and enjoy food they way people are in some other countries. This was what the book *French Women Don't Get Fat: The Secret of Eating for Pleasure* was all about. The French make time to appreciate their meals and indulge in the pleasure of good food and wine. There is no feeling of angst, guilt, deprivation or pressure to diet — or there didn't use to be. So they can eat to the point of satisfaction, knowing that another wonderful meal awaits them when they get hungry again.

If you've been raised in a culture of dieting or deprivation, you don't have the assurance that a guilt-free yummy meal awaits you. Add to that a frenzied lifestyle and you have even less assurance that any meal awaits you at all. Eating is now something that gets squeezed in between other priorities and often done on the run or out of a box, can or bag. As one of my clients remarked, "I'm lucky if I can get in one home-cooked meal a week. There just isn't time to plan, shop and prepare healthy meals for my family or for myself." It isn't just hard to make meals; it is getting harder to sit down and have time to eat them.

How can you enjoy your food or feel satisfied if you are eating whatever you can grab, doing two things at once or feeling rushed? You really can't. Satisfaction comes when you are focused on what you are eating, noticing how if tastes and feels, and choosing foods you find satisfying. This was the ah-ha Jacob was looking for. He had come to me wanting to eat better. He told me he tended to eat the wrong foods at the wrong time and his main issue was not planning for or sitting down for meals.

By tweaking his morning routine slightly he was able to sit down for breakfast and prepare salads for lunch, which he loved. Then instead of having three slices of pizza for lunch because it was easy, he found he was more satisfied when he had just one slice of pizza with his salad. By making it a priority and putting his focus on meals, he was soon finding time to prepare healthier foods and sitting down to enjoy them. He told me, "I'm now more conscientious of what I'm eating and of my satisfaction."

The combination of eating consciously, choosing things you enjoy and being free of emotional and mental baggage allows you to experience satisfaction. Most of us are disconnected from the experience by internal judgment and emotional distraction or by external busyness and unappealing choices.

Once Doreen started to discern which foods she actually liked and felt free to buy them instead of diet foods, she was able to enjoy her food more and stop when she was satisfied. She could even stop part way into a cookie or Dove bar and decide she was done, because she was able to really enjoy the experience and reach a feeling of satisfaction, and she knew she could have more at another time when she was hungry and wanted it again as part of a balanced meal.

My client Ginny used to have cravings in the afternoon that she filled with sweets and a glass of wine, but that never satisfied her. As she became more conscious of what she was eating, she became more satisfied and discovered that the cravings subsided and she was no longer driven to eat sweets. Bethany learned that if she just had what she wanted to eat in the first place, she would feel more satisfied and wouldn't want or even think about having dessert later on. She was able to finally stop overeating at night by satisfying herself at dinner. Diane had a similar experience. She told me, "Now that I've discovered satisfaction, I'm satisfied every night and not going to bed hungry from dieting or full from bingeing."

Many of my clients have learned that once they started to eat more balanced meals and snacks they are more satisfied than when they had just eaten carbohydrates or unhealthy foods. Daphne was amazed to find that she was much more satisfied when she had a better balance of protein in her meals, and Megan found the same thing when she added more fats. This was very freeing for Justine who found that balanced meals were much more satisfying to her. She told me in one of our sessions that, "The feeling of being satisfied is what I strive for now and balanced meals are much more satisfying than what I was doing before. I feel like I'm being good to myself when I have a full balanced meal." Michael had a similar experience and found that the more he chose healthier foods in balance, the more fulfilled he was and the longer that feeling lasted during the day.

Once you become familiar with what satisfaction feels like, you will find you become more conscious of your choices so you can continue to experience feeling satisfied. Justine was pleased to find that she started picking foods that would be satisfying quite easily. She told me, "I wanted a snack but I wasn't hungry, and I realized it would be more satisfying to wait and have a full meal. So I waited!! Another time when I went out to dinner I looked through the menu and then I closed my eyes and checked in with myself to see what I really wanted. I realized what I wanted was chicken salad and that was very satisfying and just great."

When you aren't satisfied, you will eat more. Stuart discovered that by overeating Kashi bars when he got bored with them. He still liked them and was glad to have them when he got hungry, but if he had them too often they lost their appeal. So to compensate for feeling deprived of satisfaction, he ate even more of them subconsciously. This was an important observation for him. He then understood that it mattered to him to have a variety of foods that would be satisfying. The more familiar he got with satisfaction, the more intuitive healthy eating became and the more empowered he felt.

Differentiating Physical and Emotional Hunger

As you start to gain familiarity with your hunger levels, you may find that there are times when you aren't so sure if the hunger is actually physical or perhaps something else. It is common to confuse being tired or stressed with being hungry or to associate cravings with hunger.

As you get to know your physical sensations of hunger, you can check in with yourself to see which of them are present when you think you are hungry. If you get a gnawing sensation as I do, check and see if you are experiencing that sensation. If not, what sensation do you have and what might it represent? A drop in energy, for example, is not always tied to hunger. Although for diabetics it may be a signal their blood sugars are dropping too low and they need food immediately. It is important to first recognize how your body registers hunger, and from that knowledge you can tell if you are getting a different type of sensation.

Roger realized he drank a bit too much and overate when he got home from a long day at work. He had thought he was super hungry, but it was actually the feeling of being spent and giving all of himself to others during the day. What he really needed was some down time to get rejuvenated after work, a way to release the built-up tension of the day, and an outlet for his feelings.

Ginny discovered she ate when she was stressed or tired, thinking it would make her feel better even though it never did. "I'm now checking in with my hunger to see if I'm really hungry or not," Ginny explained to me in our third session. "I'm finding that when I feel tired and want to eat that it works to ask myself if I am hungry and what is really going on." Doreen and Carmen had a different experience with feeling tired or exhausted by stress and would eat past the point of satisfaction into extreme fullness.

When Annette started to pay more attention to her sugar cravings, she found that she wasn't actually hungry but bored, tired, low in energy or pre-menstrual. Lucy's insight came while watching TV and seeing people eat nachos with cheese. She thought it was hunger that led her into the kitchen to make some for herself, but she then realized she wasn't actually hungry at all. She was driven into the kitchen by wanting what they had. For Stuart, what he initially thought was hunger was actually an attempt to self-medicate and increase his energy.

It can take time to really separate emotional from physical hunger, yet I find many people do make the distinction within the first few weeks if they have experiences that help them to be observant. Not everyone has frequent enough emotional hunger experiences to catch the sensations right away. Just be aware that there may be times when you assume you are hungry, only to find out that you've had more food than you need. That's okay. When that happens you get another opportunity to learn more about yourself and your body.

Achieving Portion Control Effortlessly

The hunger scale is a powerful tool that helps you determine when and how much to eat. It is also the best mechanism for managing your appetite and controlling your portions. You don't need pills to suppress your appetite or calorie counting to govern your quantities if you pay attention to your hunger levels. You can put your trust in these signals, which are generated by hormones that govern your digestion, metabolism and blood sugars, and your intuition to guide you correctly in knowing how much to eat to support your body.

If you eat a balanced meal when you are hungry and stop when you are satisfied, you will get the perfect amount of food to fill your stomach and carry you for a few hours. Initially when you first start eating according to your hunger levels, you will be experimenting to see how much food that really takes. Before you know it, you will find you start to eat most of your meals starting at a 2 and ending around a 7. This narrows down which meals or snacks are being impacted by something other than hunger, which makes it easier to focus your attention on those events.

When Irene first started using the hunger scale, she found that it made her more aware of portion sizes than she'd been in the past and she could easily do it without it being a big deal. The more she got the hang of her hunger levels and found ways to check in as she ate, the more she saw it really did provide a simple governing tool for portion control. Monica loved the scale and said, "It feels liberating to figure this out. I am eating plenty of food without counting points." Just by listening to her body she intuitively gave herself better portions. The big test was at Thanksgiving when she normally eats too much. She was able to leave half the food on her plate and save room for dessert without getting full. She paid attention and knew to stop in time and was satisfied without over doing it.

The trick is checking in with yourself as you eat and stopping before you get full, which is challenging at first. There is no physical sensation once you start eating that indicates you've had enough or obvious cues that remind you to check in. So you have to be a bit creative and try different strategies to see what works for you. Irene did pretty well at home, but when she ate with other people she got distracted and forgot all about it. She needed a visual reminder that she could easily see on her hands or on the table, and she came up with the idea to wear a ring that she only wore on these occasions. Since she didn't usually wear the ring, she would notice it on her finger more easily, and this seemed to work. Another client decided to place a key ring I had given her with my logo on the table, which reminded her of our coaching calls and to check in with herself throughout the meal.

Roger's approach was to eat about two-thirds of what was on his dinner plate and then push the plate a bit further away from himself as a symbolic gesture. It worked to get his attention and helped him decide if he really wanted more. Bethany learned her limits by looking at the food on her plate and determining what would be half and stopping when she reached that point. If she wanted more, she would again stop half way with what was left and see if she wanted to finish it off.

Patricia, like many other clients, found stopping when satisfied particularly hard because she was a "plate-cleaner". She had been raised to eat everything on her plate and didn't seem to be able to stop. As a result, she wasn't in control of how much she ate; instead the plate was in control. Patricia needed to change her belief she was a plate-cleaner. To do that, I asked her to leave something on her plate when she ate. If she was still hungry she could get more food, but she needed to show herself at an subconscious level that she was no longer a plate-cleaner. Soon she was finding it easier to leave food and being more in touch with what felt good.

Gabriella had a similar issue and realized she was determining fullness based on when her plate was empty, not on how she felt. She decided to use smaller bowls and plates or take smaller portions to begin with and then determine if she wanted more. Her other strategy was to take home half of her food when she ate out and have it for lunch the next day, and if she was still hungry when she got home she could get a little something more to eat. Both strategies helped enormously in changing her eating patterns.

Michael traveled a lot and didn't have a place to store extra food. He overate most nights, eating everything he was served so the meal wouldn't go to waste and to be sure he wouldn't get hungry later on when there was no access to food. Once he realized what was driving him to eat so much, he decided to start asking for smaller portions. When that wasn't possible, he decided it was okay to let the food be thrown away if he didn't finish it. Back in his room, he had some food bars and fruit that he always brought on his trips in case he did get hungry later on. He got very clear that he was happier being satisfied and eating less at dinner than putting the extra food on his waist.

The issue for Annette and Jacob was more challenging because they were cooks and tasted food all day. They seldom sat down to a meal or ate enough to get them from a 2 to a 7 on the hunger scale. So they both had to shift their thinking and make it a point to taste less and sit down to meals more often. When they changed their habits, they were able to see how much food they really needed and gained an understanding of appropriate portions. "My portion sizes are now more in line," Jacob told me. "My eating is more manageable and I can now tell how much is satisfying and enough. I'm no longer finishing everything on my plate because it is there, and I'm not putting so much on my plate to begin with. I'm amazed how much less I'm eating and have no desire to eat as I was before. This really suits me and I feel like I've fallen into a good zone."

By the way, your hunger levels adjust to your metabolic rates and increased need for food. If you become more active, you will be hungrier. If your metabolic rate increases, you will need to eat more food before reaching a 7 and you may be hungrier more often. And if you get pregnant (ladies), you will need to eat just a bit more to reach a 7 when you shift into the second trimester and again in the third. Your body really does know how much food you need and when.

Using a Discovery Journal

The second tool I want to introduce you to is the discovery journal. The best way to be in touch with your hunger levels and stay conscious of them regularly is to have a place to record what you are feeling. This journal is not like any other food journal you have seen or used before because the emphasis is not on tracking specific foods or calories.

It is instead a consciousness-raising journal that emphasizes your hunger levels, when you eat, and your thoughts and feelings. It is not used to judge what, when or how much you ate. It doesn't track your food intake against a set of rules. It gives you a way to be conscious and make discoveries about your eating behaviors so you can have curiosity about what might be happening. When you overeat, for example, simply say to yourself, "Isn't that interesting, I'm getting full." or "Isn't it interesting, I can't seem to stop."

If you are feeling judged for what or how much you ate, you can't be a neutral observer or ask yourself why it is that you might have overeaten, denied your hunger or felt compelled to eat when you weren't hungry. And these are questions you want to feel safe asking yourself and understanding.

On the next page is a sample discovery journal sheet for one day. You can see there is a place to keep track of the date and day of week at the top, and then along the left side a place for the times when you eat. The times will become more important as you start to keep your own journal because you will begin to notice if and when you eat every 3-4 hours or if there are much shorter or longer periods of time between eating.

Name:	Date:	M T W TH F Sa Su											
						Hunger Scale							
Time	Meal	0	1	2	3	4	5	6	7	8	9	10	Mood - Thoughts - Feelings
	Breakfast			X					X				
	Snack												
	Lunch												
	Snack												
	Dinner												

You can also see that you won't be writing down the foods you eat, at least not initially. Instead you will be indicating what type of meal you are eating. You will also note where you are on the hunger scale when you start eating and when you stop. So there will be two marks, which I show as an x. In this example, the person began eating breakfast when they were hungry at a 2 and stopped when they were satisfied at a 7, before getting full.

The largest area in this journal is for writing down thoughts, feelings or anything you are feeling physically. It is a place for writing anything that seems noteworthy or describes what was happening at the time. You will be amazed by the insights you will get from writing things down, no matter how insignificant they may seem at the time.

Here's an example from Michael's journal during his first week. He discovered it was best to write things down as soon after eating as he could, otherwise he didn't remember later in the day what his hunger levels were or what was going on at the time.

Name: Michael	Date: 4/2	M T W TH F Sa Su												
		Hunger Scale												
Time	Meal	0	1	2	3	4	5	6	7	8	9	10	Mood - Thoughts - Feelings
7:30am	Breakfast				X		X						Not hungry, grabbing something on the way out the door.
10:20am	Snack		X			X							Realized was really hungry, but didn't have much to eat with me.
12:45pm	Lunch	X								X			I am super hungry, so I went out for lunch and kind of overdid it. Also annoyed with my co-worker who dropped the ball this morning and left me with the problem.
2:30pm	Snack				X			X					Needed something to eat. Not having a good day.
7:30pm	Dinner		X							X			Hungry and had one of my favorite meals and just couldn't stop.
8:45	Snack						X			X			I have a sweet tooth, just like my dad. I always have to have sweets at night.

What you notice from his journal on Wednesday is that he is becoming aware of his hunger levels and that he seldom eats when he's hungry or stops when he gets full. His eating is all over the map and seldom driven by his physical hunger levels. This is not a judgment; it is an observation.

You can also start to get some insight about what is driving his eating behaviors by what he's written down about his day. In the morning, he hasn't allowed time to eat so this is an opportunity to look at ways where he can schedule in breakfast. Because he hasn't eaten enough, he is understandably quite hungry three hours later. Since he hasn't anticipated this, he again doesn't have enough food to eat to support his physical need for food. So by the time he gets some lunch he is ravenous.

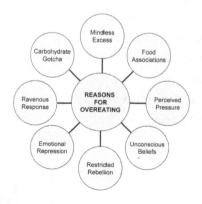

As you recall from part 2 (page 39), one of the eight reasons people overeat is a Ravenous Response. If you are that hungry, you physically and emotionally can't seem to get enough to eat and will feel compelled to overeat.

In addition, if you are repressing a feeling, such as being annoyed with someone and unable to tell them, you will have Emotional Repression and may turn to food as a coping mechanism. This often leads to overeating.

So it isn't surprising Michael overate when he finally got lunch. Rather than feeling badly about that choice, he can choose to be curious about the dynamics that led to overeating at lunch.

Less than two hours after that lunch he had a snack. The need isn't physical because he isn't hungry. It is something else, and his observation that he isn't having a good day is an opportunity to investigate if he is turning to food to deal with his frustrations.

Five hours later he's having dinner, which is a long time between meals, so not surprisingly he's pretty hungry. Not only that, he's eating one of his favorite meals. The reason he overate may be because of his Ravenous Response or because he isn't sure when he'll get to have this meal again and be experiencing a feeling of deprivation that shows up as Restricted Rebellion. He could also have been unaware at the time and overate out of Mindless Excess.

Only when I asked him more questions about his feelings, and dug a bit deeper, was he able to really see what was going on. He began getting more insights about what was driving his eating behaviors. By taking the focus off of the food, and whether he was making the right or wrong choice, he could focus on the real issue.

He started getting in touch with how his body felt and discovered he didn't enjoy how it felt to overeat, even though he did it four times on this day and frequently on other days of the week. He had no idea he overate so often. It was eye-opening for him, and he found the journaling process to be a great way to consciously and objectively see his own behaviors.

Michael didn't have a problem when I asked him to fill in the journal for me, but many people immediately resist it. Roger didn't want to journal because he believed it was associated with judgment. Sharon hated journaling and writing about her eating, and Clarissa didn't want to be so aware of her behaviors. Yet they, and others who had similar reactions, agreed to give it a try when I reassured them that there would be no judgment and they could journal as much or as little as they wanted. I also told them they could create other ways of journaling if the format didn't work for them. The objective isn't to force a specific structure on you, but to provide a tool to use in any way that works best.

Roger had some incredible insights when he filled out the journal and got more insights about his nightly routine that contributed to overeating. Sharon came to see that the journal helped her find the answer to her food issues. As she heightened her awareness about making food choices, she had less need to journal regularly. And Justine had a love-hate relationship with her journaling. Some times she saw value in using it and other times the journaling simply represented control and judgment. Yet this in and of itself is interesting. The reaction to journaling is just as much an opportunity to understand yourself as your reaction to being around food.

The discovery journal is not meant to feel like an albatross or a heavy burden, nor is it something you really need to do very often after the first couple of months. It is something that initially helps you gain greater eating consciousness, offers you insight about your eating patterns, and gives you understanding of what is subconsciously driving your behaviors. Then after using the journal for about eight weeks (when people get the most benefit), you may determine that you only want to do it when you start to feel you've lost consciousness, are having days when you are not eating well, or you are reverting back to old behaviors.

The journal is a tool to use in the way that best serves you. My only advice is to try it and give it at least four weeks to understand why it is invaluable in changing your mindset and behaviors. It is normal to feel some initial resistance or feel the diet mentality kick in, and when that happens the best thing is to keep journaling and let the beliefs and feelings come up so you can see where they are coming from and address them. You can also give yourself permission to journal on your own terms. The goal isn't to force you to journal. It is to give you a tool to help yourself in anyway that supports you, and generally it takes a couple of weeks to get the hang of it and see the power of it.

When you get past your reactions to the journal (which by the way may come and go), you will be amazed by what you learn about yourself and the amount of insight you receive. The longer you use the journal, the more opportunities you have to experience all the different types of situations where food choices are challenging for you.

As I tell my clients who feel embarrassed or upset when they have to write down a challenging situation they succumbed to, I remind them that this is actually ideal. You want to experience your most challenging moments while you are journaling because it will likely happen again. You can then uncover the root of the issue and create a strategy that can be used the next time it presents itself. See it is a blessing instead of a curse. Better yet, see it as a gift and the answer you've been waiting for. Most of my clients now do.

Patricia found the journaling helped her to stay focused, see how often she did eat well, and pinpoint where it was in her day that she struggled the most and why. Karl used it to observe and learn about what led him to overeat or choose foods that affected his glucose levels, while Ginny found it helpful to figure out how to deal with situations where she didn't feel so in control. Lucy didn't find the journaling easy, but she stuck with it and realized she didn't eat enough to ever feel satisfied and let herself get ravenous on a regular basis. It became obvious to her that she was stuck in the diet mentality. The more she used the journal, the more she took care of herself, ate enough food, and understood what was driving her to overeat at night.

Stuart didn't think he could journal because of his Attention Deficit Disorder (ADD). He soon discovered the inability to fill in forms was a limiting belief and an excuse as he came to appreciate that journaling is an exploration and loaded with valuable information. When he traveled on business he became anxious about doing the journal on the road. I explained there was no rule he had to journal all the time or when he went on trips and suggested he give himself permission to not do it. He discovered that he maintained his awareness and made good choices for himself. Because he had the option to let the journaling go and let it just be a part of him, he didn't have to deal with any guilt or resistance. His not dealing with guilt allowed him to stay engaged in the process and he was pleased with the results. He decided to create his own form for journaling that worked well for him.

I do want to point out that after the first week or so of writing down what you are experiencing with food and getting more conscious, some find they are overly conscious and have anxiety about having so much food awareness. "Being conscious and journaling feels like a diet," said Clarissa a few weeks into the process. "Being unconscious means I can do whatever I want." I promise you that this passes, as it did for Clarissa. It is normal to feel hyper-vigilant at first, but that is just part of the newness of it all and the unique experience of being conscious for the first time. It also tends to trigger the inner diet mentality voices, and they become an opportunity to identify the beliefs and feelings that have a hold on you and to address them.

Noticing When You Eat

As you could see from Michael's journal, he ate within two hours after lunch and then waited five hours before having dinner, and that information provided insights. As you start to use your own journal, notice the amount of time between meals and snacks.

- If you don't eat for many hours, is it possible you ignored your hunger signal?

- If you just ate and want to eat again, is that because you are physically hungry again, you didn't get enough to eat earlier or you only had simple carbohydrates that digested really fast?
- Based on what you learn, what will work better for you?

Take notice of your daily patterns and see if you are eating at specific times because that is just what you do or because you are actually hungry. Maggie learned that she ate by the clock because she always had breakfast before going to work, a snack when she got to work, lunch at noon, and something the moment she got home. She didn't think about. It was habitual. She had no idea if she was actually hungry until she started to pay more attention. She discovered she wasn't hungry for lunch until a bit later and didn't always need a midmorning snack. Yet somewhere she carried the idea that she was supposed to eat at all those times, so it was eye-opening to discover she could eat when she was actually hungry and not at any predetermined set times.

Clarissa, as well as many of my other clients, overate frequently at night because she was starving by the time she had dinner. She prided herself on being good and not eating too much during the day. Yet she learned that eating enough during the day eliminated overeating at night. Jill simply forgot to eat during the day and found when she didn't miss meals she didn't overeat later on. Tiffany as well as my client George generally skipped lunch, but discovered lunch fulfilled them and reduced their cravings for junk food later on.

Maria didn't make time to eat until she got done with work in the evening. She was always on the run and just couldn't seem to find time to eat. Yet as she began to eat breakfast more often, and then eat three meals during the day she found she felt so much better. They all learned by observing when they did and didn't eat that when monitoring their hunger levels they felt better and stopped overcompensating in the evenings or at other times by eating only when they were hungry.

Gabriella's situation was a bit different. She didn't like to eat breakfast and never felt hungry until late morning, and even then she didn't feel like eating much. So by the time she had lunch in the early afternoon she was famished and over did it. If she did have breakfast, she would skip the midmorning snack and would eat around 2 pm. She just didn't stop to notice her hunger while she was working unless it was screaming to get her attention, yet when she set an alarm to check in with herself midmorning she often found that she was in fact hungry. She was dealing with a couple of issues. She wasn't hungry first thing in the morning nor did she like the way her breakfast left her feeling, and she hated to stop working to go upstairs to eat. By the time she did get some lunch she grabbed what was fastest, not the salad she really wanted that was healthier. The same happened at dinner. She would be so hungry when she finally started making it, she would snack on crackers or overeat when she and her husband had their meal.

She isn't alone in resisting breakfast or not feeling hungry then, yet breakfast is necessary to fuel our morning metabolism and provide energy. I encouraged her, as I do others, to find something balanced to eat in the morning. It doesn't have to be much. Gabriella experimented with various foods that were appealing to her and found a whole grain cracker with cottage cheese was just right. She also tried various snacks that she could keep at her desk so that when she was hungry around 10 am she wouldn't have to stop what she was doing to get some food. This worked and she felt relaxed enough at lunch time to make a salad and eat only what felt satisfying. She also had part of a Kashi bar from the stock she kept in her desk before leaving the office so she wasn't too hungry when she made dinner. By honoring her hunger levels, she was in more control and eating exactly what she really wanted and feeling wonderfully satisfied.

One of the toughest times of day is after dinner. Most of my clients want something about an hour or two after they eat, and once they have a little something it is often hard to stop. This was when Michael always grabbed something sweet, even though he wasn't hungry, and he isn't alone. This is worth observing and understanding. If it isn't physical hunger, than what do you really want? Sometimes it is to have something sweet, and if that is the case it is best to have that with dinner. Eating dessert as part of a balanced meal gives you the satisfaction you are looking for and reduces the need to overeat or going looking for it later.

Focusing on How You Feel

As you journal and use the hunger scale, you will become more aware of how different foods, choices and situations affect you physically and emotionally.

You will discover that eating certain foods or excess quantities can make you feel sick, which is what Karl found when he had foods high in sugar that left him exhausted, in pain or with a raging headache. Anita saw just how nauseous and tired she got when she over ate junk food while traveling with her family. She told me, "I can see that what I put in my body is affecting my energy levels and how I feel physically. This experience is motivating me to change the way I eat."

Stuart also saw a direct correlation of physical symptoms whenever he ate foods high in saturated fats or that were highly processed. He said, "I just don't feel well when I eat certain foods or overeat," a couple of weeks after he started to be conscious of his body when he ate. The more he observed, the more discerning he became as to what didn't sit well with him, such as chocolate. He learned that most chocolate upset his stomach but that a specific type in small amounts was just fine.

Soon he was gravitating toward foods that made him feel better, which were a combination of complex carbohydrates, unsaturated fats and lean proteins – all of which are healthier foods – and these were easier on his digestive system. By the fifth week he was getting clearer on what felt good and what didn't and was no longer willing to pay the price of eating foods that made him feel sick. He also learned that when he needed energy the worst things to have were caffeine and simple carbohydrates. Instead he discovered that a balanced healthy snack of nuts and wholegrain crackers, some green tea and fresh air were the answer to getting re-energized.

Georgette struggled with sugar cravings and began to see she wasn't tolerating fruit very well. Right after eating an apple she crashed, and she noticed this happened frequently when she had other foods high in sugar or other simple carbohydrates. As she experimented, she began to notice that when she ate more protein and whole grains in the morning instead of a breakfast that was mostly carbohydrates (and much of it simple carbohydrates) she didn't crash so much during the day. Once she found out she had Reactive Hypoglycemia, she began eating more complex carbohydrates and balancing them with protein and unsaturated fat, which stopped the cravings. Now she is highly conscious of eating in balance and feels more energized and sane. She told me, "Now I have stopped the cycle. I don't crave sugar like I did, and I know it had nothing to do with willpower. It has to do with eating in balance to prevent the crash." Whenever she does have a crash, she immediately checks back to see what triggered it and double checks she is eating a balanced combination of protein, fat and complex carbohydrates.

Once you see which foods leave you feeling better, you will naturally gravitate toward having more of them. It will be your choice and you won't be doing it because you are supposed to but because you want to, and then the more often you choose healthier things the more you will want them. Many of my clients start to find, to their amazement, they want more fruits and vegetables and less cookies and ice cream, without any suggestion from me to change their foods.

Having a craving for vegetables is not the only thing that often surprises people; many are shocked to discover that foods they thought they loved they actually don't really care for. Abigail was really surprised to find that when she ate whatever she wanted she didn't actually enjoy it. She was getting in tune with the experience of how specific foods and eating really felt to her, and it wasn't as pleasant as she assumed. Simone and Doreen both discovered that the cookies they thought they loved so much weren't actually all that great, and Maggie found that the Pepsi she couldn't get enough of really didn't taste that good.

It isn't just the physical sensations and experience that you will start to notice. You will also start to see connections to how you feel emotionally when you eat. Henry saw almost immediately that whenever he was annoyed he had to cool off with a beer and something to eat and that he was seldom all that thirsty or hungry when this happened. Justine began to distinguish between real hunger and cravings, and then had a huge realization that she only got cravings when she was anxious, unhappy, depressed or felt guilty for not getting something done. She could see that her emotions were driving her cravings.

Maggie had her own epiphany when she finally understood it really wasn't about the food she ate to control her feelings or deal with her stress, and that it was okay to feel the pain, face her doubts and let out her emotions. She told me, "I think this was the first time in my life that I actually tried to feel the emotion and not eat it away. I forgot all about the food within five minutes. It was amazing to just sit and think about what was really going on and not eat out of emotion."

For Lucy, she didn't just notice how she felt when she ate but she noticed how she felt throughout the day and realized that she was irritated, worried, stressed and always felt like she was racing. She also noticed she was continually starving in the morning, eating on the run and not getting enough food during the day and starving again when she got home at night. Being hungry and wanting comfort then drove her to overeat most nights of the week. Daphne also zeroed in on how she was feeling during the day and discovered she felt overwhelmed by the demands on her time. As a wife, mother of three, self-employed business woman and daughter of aging parents in need of support, she realized she had stopped taking care of herself and was craving sugar to get through the day. The insight they both got helped them examine what they needed to do to reduce the stress in their lives and get more time to eat and breathe.

Appreciating Conscious Awareness

An amazing thing happens when you choose to be aware of what you are doing, eating and feeling, and that is you want to remain conscious. You come to value your ability to observe, understand and make choices that feel better.

Most people find that once they experience what it really feels like to be hungry and full, to be sick from overeating or eating unhealthy things, or to be driven to eat by subconscious emotions or beliefs that something in them changes and they never go back to what they were doing before. It isn't always as simple as that, but a fundamental shift does happen by gaining a conscious awareness of what you feel when eating, and a part of you doesn't want to go back to what you were doing before.

Many of my clients come up with their own way of journaling so they can regain consciousness when it slips, using an approach that best fits their personality and lifestyle. Some use little notebooks or find ways to fit a week of meals on a page. I encourage you to devise your own method after a couple of weeks of using the journal pages (see the appendix to get copies from me at no cost), so that you are more inclined to use it or turn to it when you need to recapture your awareness or see what is driving you to make uncomfortable choices.

For some people gaining awareness is all it takes to change their behaviors and eat healthier. But for most there is more to it, and their consciousness without judgment becomes the foundation and the first C for understanding what is triggering their behaviors and making healthier choices.

Coaching Questions to
GET STARTED CONSCIOUSLY

What does hunger feel like for you?

How do you know when you are getting full?

What helps you know that you are satisfied?

What patterns do you observe about your eating behaviors as you start using the hunger scale and journal?

When are you eating, and how often is it because you are physically hungry?

What do you notice about the times you go for food and you aren't hungry?

What do you notice about the times you overeat?

How does the way you eat, or what you eat, feel to you physically?

Understanding What Drives Your Behaviors

Now that you are becoming more aware of your own eating behaviors and getting curious about why you may be overeating, under eating or eating for no apparent reason at all, the next step is to dig a bit deeper to find out more. As you now know, what is really going on isn't always cut and dry. There are lots of different reasons that could be driving you to make the choices you do, and most of them are subconscious.

As I often remind clients, it is more important to know why you are eating too much or turning to food than it is to have not been able to stop yourself. You can't always stop, and if you think you should have been able to leads to self-criticism and self-doubt. Okay, so you ate it or had more than you really wanted. Why might that be? What drove you to eat something you didn't need physically and probably didn't even enjoy? That is what you want to focus on. That is the key.

When you finally understand what is triggering you, you will stop sooner or not even turn to food in the first place. The important thing is not to beat yourself up if you find yourself eating when you didn't mean to. This is a journey and the process doesn't happen over night. It takes weeks, and for some people months of getting to know themselves and then changing their thinking, routines and dealing with the source of their beliefs and emotions. You didn't get to the place you are at now overnight, so don't expect immediate changes.

Let's go back to what drives behaviors in the first place, which I covered in part 2.

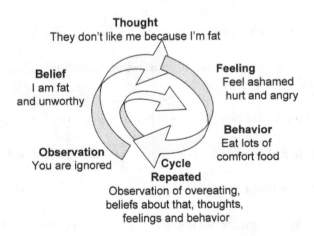

Most behaviors are choices that are driven by underlying beliefs and feelings, yet what you are more aware of is what you did or didn't do and the judgment that follows. Most people harshly judge themselves for their behaviors without understanding that the behavior has nothing to do with them being good or bad. First of all, we are not our behaviors. We may have a bad behavior, but that doesn't make us bad. Furthermore, few of us deliberately set out to behave badly. So when you overeat and then judge yourself harshly for being bad, you are accusing yourself of deliberately doing a bad thing as if you meant to cause yourself harm. Obviously that isn't the case. More importantly, the behavior isn't about being bad or good. It is about the underlying drivers that led to that moment and your belief that it is bad.

I first came to understand the role of beliefs and feelings from Diana Lipson-Burge RD, who I studied with to become certified as an intuitive and emotional eating coach and who co-authored *Un-Dieting: Un-Doing the Diet Mentality*.

Thoughts validate what you've been taught to believe about yourself and your world. Those beliefs come from your family, friends, schooling and society. Beliefs about food come from what you experienced at home, all the diets you've read about or tried, the news and shows you've watched promoting specific diet approaches, and what you see in magazines that offer quick ways to lose weight alongside pictures of beautifully thin women and yummy desserts.

What most people believe after years of exposure to these messages and trying to succeed with various diets and weight loss programs is: all the yummy foods are bad for you, only thin people can eat the good stuff, the best way to be in control is to avoid having forbidden foods in the house, it is best to suppress your hunger and avoid eating whenever you can, all it takes is more willpower, its impossible to stick with a diet, if you can't be good then you are bad, and it is hopeless. Some also believe they are sugar addicts, worthless, and never going to lose weight so why bother even trying.

These beliefs are negative, judgmental and go against what you would want to believe for yourself. Yet they are reinforced by the parental thoughts in your head that incessantly tries to keep you in line with the dogma it knows. If you wrote down all your beliefs about food and eating, as I have, you would be shocked by what you've taken on as the doctrine for your life. The good news is you don't have to keep these beliefs. Once you know what they are, you can change them into empowering positive beliefs that support you in realistic encouraging ways. The more often you state your new affirmations and remind yourself of your new beliefs, the more you dampen the old ones and the inner self-critic.

Beliefs don't just drive your thoughts; they also impact how you feel and whether it is safe to express those feelings or get your needs met. The more rigid and restrictive your beliefs, the more you are holding yourself back and repressing your feelings. If your beliefs are based on high standards, perfectionism and your inability to please others enough for example, you will likely feel unworthy, incompetent and ashamed. These are not good feelings, yet they are valid and have a right to be expressed. In fact, the more you push them away, the more entrenched they become in your body and psyche and show up in things like overeating, shopping, workaholism, passive-aggressive behavior and addictions.

By allowing the feelings to be validated, expressed and understood, you release the burden and have an opportunity to address what led to these feelings in the first place: your unmet needs. Those needs are represented by that other set of thoughts from the deprived child that rises up and rebels against the enforcer, claiming it can have what it wants.

The *I am feeling or I am thinking... because...* process I introduced you to in part 2 is incredibly powerful in helping you understand your feelings and beliefs and determining your unmet needs. Once you get in touch with your inner voices, understand what you need, why you need it and how to resolve it, then you can more easily identify what your urges for food are all about and make a conscious choice to address the real need instead of covering it up or placating an old belief or feeling.

While I have emphasized how beliefs, thoughts and feelings drive your behaviors around food, there are a number of other things that can impact your behaviors as I've mentioned before. Don't assume that every time you eat outside of the hunger scale it is because of subconscious beliefs or emotions because that isn't necessarily the case.

Getting Clues from Journaling

When you first start journaling, you may notice most of the thoughts and feelings you've written about are cursory, such as "Enjoyed my lunch"; "Probably over did it"; "In a rush"; Not feeling all that well"; "Having a bad day" or "Whatever." These comments describe what is happening at a surface level, yet mostly likely there is much more beneath these comments.

Now that you have a better understanding of what drives eating behaviors, I encourage you to write more about the thoughts and feelings you experience when you eat. These additional comments can give you better insight as to what is or was driving your choices. Be honest with yourself and explore specific situations, events or patterns when you didn't eat when you were hungry, kept eating past the point of satisfaction, or ate things that didn't feel good to your body.

Anything you write down can give you clues, even if you don't think so at the time. Irene noted that the eggnog she had one afternoon while shopping was free. She wasn't hungry and she had a large cup of it, which left her feeling uncomfortable. Was getting something free hard to say no to? Was this possibly tied to a belief that you don't turn down something free or a good deal? Was there also a belief she couldn't throw out some of the eggnog because the person that gave it to her was looking on?

Many people feel they can't pass up a good deal or be rude by having just a tiny bit of something offered them, so they have more than they want. Yet a good deal isn't so good if you don't need it, and it is not rude to say no thanks or thanks this is all I want. For Irene, what was really going on was she loves eggnog and knew she wouldn't get more, which created a feeling of deprivation and the desire to get as much as she could while it was there. The reason isn't always obvious, so ask yourself a number of questions to narrow it down.

Bethany had eaten way past the point of full at dinner and wrote, "Out with friends – not my pick of a restaurant" in her journal. Was she simply distracted or irritated? She realized it was a bit of both. She was simply not in touch with her hunger levels or her feelings and she wanted a way to be more conscious. What would help her do that? She considered wearing a bracelet when out but instead determined the best thing was to decide ahead of time where in the meal she would stop and check in.

Another time she ate an entire sandwich for lunch and felt awful afterward. She was at work and noted, "I might get hungry later if didn't finish it." Couldn't she eat just part of it and have more if she did get hungry later in the afternoon? Was there a reason she couldn't do that? It wasn't a problem to take a break and eat more later on, but she had a belief she had to eat it all at once. Where did that belief come from? Did she gain something by having this belief? Could she change this belief so she had more options? She realized how silly it was to believe she had to eat more than enough just in case she couldn't get more food, and did change it. She was then able to enjoy the flexibility of eating only what she needed and having more if she got hungry again. She was thrilled by how well this worked for her. She was no longer stuffed after lunch and felt so much better and at ease.

Gail had a week of skipping meals, overeating and choosing foods that didn't leave her feeling very well. Her journal entries were "No food in the house"; "Getting to bed too late" and "Letting work be the priority." Was this a scheduling problem or something more? How did it feel that she wasn't able to put her health and needs first? How could she get healthier foods prepared in advance for when she got hungry? She saw that it was a matter of putting herself first and making time on the weekends to plan, shop and prepare foods for the week. The more she did this, the better she felt physically and about herself.

Anita often put in her journal "While baby ate"; "In car" and "On way home from grocery store." She was a new mother and learning how to put herself first. These entries helped her see that she wasn't taking time out to eat when she was hungry or setting aside time to eat a well-balanced meal. Instead she was eating what her son didn't finish, snacking on foods that weren't healthy and eating late dinners with her husband. This wasn't helping her reach her goals. She decided to make time for breakfast in the morning and suggested eating earlier at night to her husband so her family could have a healthy meal together. She also looked for healthy snack alternatives for those times when she had to eat on the run. As she did this, she had a sense of accomplishment and was enjoying healthier meals.

Many people discover from journaling they overeat while watching TV. They are focused on what they are watching and eat everything they bring to the couch, only to discover they are way past full when their shows are over. Gabriella noticed this wasn't the only time she overate subconsciously. She saw from journaling that it happened while having conversations, drinking wine, feeling tired or being angry. This insight helped her create some strategies to be more aware of how much was eating and to stop sooner.

Clarissa also discovered in her journal that she did mindless eating while going through emails or while watching TV, and her solution was to stop having food around while doing these things. She also kept writing "bored" in her notes. She hadn't known the extent that she was bored until she saw this. This opened her mind to ask, what would be less boring to eat or do? What did she really enjoy and need?

Simone, like so many people, wanted something sweet at night an hour or so after dinner. She wrote the second week of keeping a journal, "Stressed about going back to work tomorrow." She was seeing a pattern of stress eating and in the fourth week of journaling she knew why she was craving something on a Sunday night and chose to address it. She noted in her journal, "Want something sweet. Instead I decided to plan my week, which made me feel better." She had learned from journaling what was triggering her and how to help herself address the underlying issue.

When Karl ate a lot of pretzels he wrote, "I need something to crunch on." What else did he want to crunch on? Can you pick up that there is possibly some irritation or emotion hiding behind this comment? Cindy wrote, "Good" when she felt that she'd eaten the right things and stopped before reaching full, and then when she had a lot for a late night dessert she put down "Oops, bad but didn't care at the time." Is her diet mentality enforcer still governing her? Was she feeling so judged about the dessert that she pushed the feelings away? How was she really feeling when she had dessert and what deeper feelings are tied to that?

Listening to Your Internal Voices

Cindy's "good" and "bad" judgment comes from the enforcer of her belief system, while the "but didn't care at the time" was from her deprived child, as I discussed earlier in this section. The more the enforcer beats her up for not doing what she should, the less the child wants to hear about it and acts out by doing what it wants despite the consequences. Outwardly the consequences show up on the scale and in your clothes, but these are not as damaging as what happens inwardly where your self-esteem is further eroded and the battle rages on and the stakes get higher for control. They may also involve other voices to support them in gaining the upper hand — much like the enforcer rallies the support of the critic.

Our inner voices are sub-personalities of our ego. I've primarily focused on two of them: the enforcer and deprived child, but there are many more. Some of them may also be playing a role in your food behaviors. One of the foremost practitioners of Voice Dialog is Tim Kelley who co-authored *Wake Up…Live the Life You Love: Living on Purpose*. I have been fortunate to know and learn from him. He has helped me to identify the protector, critic, image consultant, skeptic and wounded child, among others, and he says there are hundreds of these voices in each of us. We don't all have the same voices in our persona, and the voices we do have may choose to go by different names.

Stuart discovered he had a committee of voices involved in his food behaviors. He quickly identified the voice of his enforcer, who he associated with his mother and how she dictated what he would or wouldn't eat and restricted access to the foods he loved so much. He also recognized the deprived child that couldn't get enough, who he called the indulger. They were in a constant battle, which drove him to overeat and choose snack foods that continually made him sick.

By adding a third voice that he called the neutral observer, the other voices began to calm down. The neutral observer kept an eye on his hunger levels, listened to how his body felt and helped him see when the enforcer and indulger were being triggered. He could see when the indulger took over in the afternoon and wanted snack foods, and by doing the "*I am feeling … because …*" inquiry he began to understand what the indulger really needed and how to address those needs.

In just six weeks he told me, "The enforcer and indulger have reached a truce," and Stuart was then able to meet both of their needs without repressing them. One thing he learned is the indulger didn't always want food. Sometimes it wanted to be rewarded by going outside for fifteen minutes during the day. I encouraged him to return to journaling anytime he noticed that one or both the voices weren't getting their needs met so he could identify the trigger and find a resolution.

Clarissa felt certain her enforcer was really the dictator and her rebelling child the wild child, and her wild child didn't like the scrutiny that came with journaling or awareness. She had been put on a diet when she was just twelve and had been scrutinized for her food choices by a mother who perpetually dieted. Then when she married, she was scrutinized by her father-in-law whenever they ate meals with him. No wonder the wild child hated the whole idea of focusing on food and keeping track of it. What calmed this voice down was being told that Clarissa didn't have to journal and she could have whatever food she wanted whenever she was hungry. The wild child also appreciated that it was being heard and was going to get more fun and variety. By being more aware of this voice, Clarissa started to take care of those needs.

Sharon didn't think she had a rebelling voice but instead a self-sabotager that was getting in the way of making healthier choices. I suggested she dialog with it and find out what it was getting by sabotaging her efforts and what it wanted. As Tim has helped me to understand, the voices aren't going away. They have a function to perform and while it may seem they aren't helping, they do in fact want what is best for us and are responding to our beliefs and our other voices. By identifying their true role and what they are trying to accomplish you can work with them to support you differently.

The inner critic was the voice making itself most known to Abigail. As she learned to be an observer, she saw ways of breaking the cycle of self-criticism by reinforcing her other voice of compassion. She did this by letting the critic know she was worthy without being perfect. She focused on being good to herself by making time for relaxation, exercise, good nutrition and rest, which the critic really wanted her to do. She also became familiar with what triggered her critic to judge her and began changing her beliefs.

The voice Gabriella discovered was similar to the deprived child. It was Poor Me, who felt sorry for itself and was in need of attention after a hard day at work, when things weren't going well or from doing more than its fair share. Once she recognized the voice, she also recognized what it really needed which was acknowledgement and empathy. As soon as she became conscious of this voice and took time to listen and validate it, she found the desire for food when she wasn't hungry vanished.

You don't have to identify specific voices to hear your own self-criticism, to know you are judging yourself, like the guy who called himself a big fat disgusting cow, or to become in touch with your needs. You will see it in your journal notes and you will start to hear it as you tune into what you say to yourself. When Christina first started to keep her discovery journal she wrote, "Will never be thin anyways" next to a time she ate a lot of sugary foods. She was putting herself down and feeling helpless, and she could see it in the words she wrote.

Barbara caught her self-critic saying she was fat and she quickly changed it to "I am wonderful, pretty and look great." She felt happy in that moment, and she was pleased that she stopped her inner judgment. If you pay attention to what you tell yourself and challenge the truthfulness of what you hear, you will be able to see yourself shift from hateful comments to more loving ones. The more you think of yourself *as if...* you are wonderful, great and beautiful or as if you are successful, capable and in control, the more you will come to believe it – even if one of your voices vehemently disagrees.

Betsy, who was obese, wanted to see what would happen by thinking she were thin for a day. "It really worked," she told me the following week. "I felt more confident, in control and good about myself when I did it." This became one of her goals to do regularly because, as she said in another session, "It so really works." As she learned, you are what you tell your ego you are, no matter if it is positive or negative. The more you say positive empowering things about yourself, even if you don't fully believe them initially, the better you feel. As you change what you think, believe and feel, you can't help but change your behaviors to match your internal mindset.

Identifying Your Beliefs & Emotions

At this point you may now have a good handle on the most obvious reasons you over or under eat, but you may still be finding yourself eating past a 7 or grabbing something when you aren't hungry. Being conscious of this or of what your internal voices are saying is one thing, addressing the underlying beliefs and feelings are another.

Many consider both beliefs and feelings drivers of emotional eating, yet I have found it is more helpful to separate beliefs from emotions and put them in a different category of "belief eating". If you believe you deserve a reward after work, for example, you will become preoccupied with getting food when your work is done. While there may be emotional attachment to the needs associated with your beliefs, the real issue is the beliefs themselves.

<u>Belief Eating</u>

There are several drivers of belief eating, which I've touched on in the eight reasons for overeating. They are food associations, subconscious beliefs and perceived pressure. In each case, your beliefs are playing a role in your behaviors around food.

Food associations

Food associations tend to pair food (sometimes specific foods) with specific scenarios, and these are created from your past experiences or what you grew up learning. They are part of your history, tradition and routines. For example, Americans always have a turkey on Thanksgiving accompanied by a feast of traditional side dishes based on family recipes and a variety of pumpkin, pecan and apple pies.

Some of the more common associations are tied to celebrations, holidays, being sick, or types of meals. For example: dinner and dessert or birthdays and cake. Sometimes they are tied to a specific food or drink, such as Oreo cookies and milk, coffee and biscotti, or apple pie and ice cream. It would seem weird not to have one without the other. One of my clients pointed out that it would be weird not to have corn on the cob, hotdogs and ice cream when summer came and that was what she looked forward to every year.

Associations can be tied to feelings, such as being happy or sad. It isn't so much that these are repressed feelings that are driving emotional eating as they are associations. If you grew up eating to celebrate and be happy as Tiffany did or you were given something to eat whenever you were sad to cheer you up, then these are hidden associations that will drive you to eat whenever the feeling occurs whether they are repressed or not. Maggie was given food to calm her down whenever she fell or got hurt, and to this day she wants food when she injures herself.

In the last section, I shared how Tiffany believed she deserved a reward after work just because she had always been rewarded for getting things done growing up. Nearly everyone I have ever worked with has discovered they have the same kind of reward association with food, which isn't surprising. Most kids get a snack when they come home from school or get rewarded with food when they are good. As a result we are programmed to desire food when we feel deserving after a hard day at work, exerting ourselves or doing something we didn't want to do.

We want validation of our efforts and a gold star, and we want the feeling that comes from the recognition and appreciation. There is nothing wrong with wanting that, and once you know this is what you need, you can look for other ways to reward yourself that don't involve food. The key is in understanding what it is that you are getting from the reward, so you can look for an alternative that fulfills that need in you. There are many ways of feeling rewarded that are just as simple and accessible as food.

Some alternatives that my clients have come up with for themselves include having a cup of really good tea, calling a good friend, taking an aromatherapy bath, enjoying the calm and taking ten minutes to breathe, going for a quick walk in the fresh air, gardening, cooking a great meal, playing with their dog or cat, listening to an uplifting song, cuddling with their spouse, taking a scenic drive home, and going to see the sunset. It helps to come up with a short list ahead of time, so you can quickly identify other accessible options besides food that will feel rewarding to you.

To determine if you have a food association with an event, situation or feeling, ask yourself when you habitually grab something automatically, what is driving you to do this?

> What are you thinking?

> What are you feeling?

If it is a food association it will most likely be a thought (instead of a feeling) and something like *I need, I want, I deserve or I have to have* _____. You want milk because you are having cookies, you have to have corn on the cob because its summer, you need food because you are happy, or you deserve a reward because you finished your work.

> I am thinking _____ because _____

If you aren't sure if this is a food association, keep digging to see where the belief comes from. Why do you need or want it? Is there an association or is it tied to something else? And what feeling do you get?

> The belief comes from _____

> The feeling I get from this is _____

Next see what else will fulfill that feeling besides food.

> What else will provide the same feeling that isn't food?
>
> _____

By asking these questions, you are getting at your thoughts, their underlying beliefs and where you got the belief from. Knowing the source of the belief can be helpful in putting it in perspective and understanding the feelings will help you identify why you may want to hold onto the belief. At some point in your life the belief may have served you well. The question now is, does it still serve you or is it holding you back from living a full and better life. If it is holding you back, you can give yourself permission to release it and replace it with a new belief that serves your best interests.

Does this belief serve you or is it holding you back from what you want?

_____

If it doesn't serve you, can you give yourself permission to release it?

_____

What new belief will better support you now?

_____

Sometimes just knowing there is an association is enough to stop this particular eating behavior because you can easily recognize what is going on. Yet more often the association is so ingrained that you have to come up with strategies to redirect your behavior each time you see the association. In time, the associations will abate or you will have new ones that are not tied to food.

Give yourself time to make the shift, and go easy on yourself. There will be times when it is quite appropriate to eat within context to the identified association because you are hungry and you planned for it. The goal is to avoid mindlessly eating food out of habitual association, whether or not you want or feel a need for the food.

Subconscious beliefs
Subconscious beliefs are governed by rules about food that we got from our families, peers or diets. These underlying rules are identifiable by the *shoulds* or *musts* in your thinking. Common subconscious beliefs about food are: you must eat everything on your plate, don't waste food because people are starving in Africa, dinner is followed by dessert, you might not get enough so it is best to eat it while you can, you shouldn't eat after 6 pm, all it takes is willpower to be in control, and if you can be good during the day you can eat more at night. No doubt you can add many more to this list, including specific foods you should and shouldn't have.

As you may recall, Tiffany had beliefs about leftovers and throwing out food that put her in a bind. She felt she had no choice but to eat any food that remained after cooking a meal. I had asked her why that was. What was she thinking at the time and why? She said, "I was thinking I have to eat this food because I can't throw it out or keep it." Where did that belief come from that she couldn't throw it out or keep it? It came from her mother.

I also asked her whether the beliefs she got from her mother were ones she wanted to keep. Were they serving her? She was an adult and could decide for herself if she wanted to keep these rules for her own household or for herself. She could see they weren't working for her, but she also knew they wouldn't be easy to give up. For her to make the changes, she created new beliefs and practiced strategies to support them. It wasn't easy for her to throw out food, so she needed to find a way to throw things out where she couldn't turn around and retrieve them a half hour later when she lost her resolve. She also needed a way to store leftovers so they wouldn't smell up her refrigerator or look unkempt, which was important to her. With some brainstorming she came up with ways to address these.

It isn't as simple as waving a magic wand and deciding to change your beliefs overnight. It takes conscious awareness to stop yourself when eating out of old thinking, remind yourself of your new belief, take action according to this belief and do it often enough that it becomes more habitual. The repetition reinforces and affirms your new beliefs and behaviors. In time, these will become natural to you.

The way Patricia stopped eating everything on her plate was to leave a little something each time. This wasn't easy to do initially but the more she did it the more it helped her replace the belief "I'm a plate-cleaner" to "I am not a plate-cleaner." It wasn't long before she believed she wasn't a plate-cleaner because each time she left something her new belief was being proven right.

Nicholas believed that if he had junk food in the house he had to finish it before eating other healthier things. In part this was tied to thinking he couldn't waste the food and it had to be eaten. His other belief was it was best to do it sooner than later to get the food out of the house so he wouldn't feel so tempted by it. He could see this was illogical, but he couldn't think any differently when the food was around him. He needed both a new belief and a strategy for having less healthy foods in the house. His new belief was "Food is more wasted in me than in the trash." His strategy for junk food was to buy it in smaller serving sizes so he had only as much as he really wanted as part of a balanced meal and the rest, which wasn't very much, could be tossed out. It worked.

He found he only wanted a few bites, and he felt fine throwing out the remainder knowing it actually cost less than if he indulged in it.

The belief that you might not get enough of something you want can come from many sources. For some of my female clients this came from growing up with a parent who limited their food in order to control their weight. For those that have dieted considerably, it comes from striving to meet dietary restrictions. And for others it can be from growing up during a war or depression or being part of a large family without enough money to keep food on the table.

When you have been severely deprived, a part of you is constantly trying to make up for what you didn't get in the past. Once you understand the source of the deprivation, you can reassure yourself that you will be able to get what you want again. This reduces the anxiety and the associated need to make up for the deprivation, which allows you to enjoy a small amount of what you really want or decide you don't even really want it right then, knowing you can have it another time. It is giving yourself permission to be fulfilled that takes the power away from the belief you are or will be deprived once again.

Another belief that has numerous sources is that it takes willpower to control yourself around food. No doubt you heard this at home, from peers and colleagues, and from dieting programs. Joellen believed if she was strict enough and hard enough on herself, she should be able to change her behaviors and be good. Yet the more she tried to enforce these rules upon herself the more often she ended up bingeing on ice cream, donuts and Dairy Queen dilly bars. This would lead to a round of retribution where she would eat only diet food and restrict herself as much as possible to re-exert control. The more she tried to gain the upper hand, the more she lost it and her self-esteem. She had to stop the judgment to see she was carrying a self-sabotaging belief and to learn that focusing on willpower wasn't the answer. The answer was allowing some slack and focusing on strategies that didn't rely on willpower at all to eat in a healthier way. The easier she was on herself, the less she binged. Her new belief was, "I eat what my body wants and needs and I don't have to control everything I do." This new belief calmed down her inner voices that used to make her crazy.

One of the best ways to address overeating dessert in the evening is to include it in with dinner as part of your balanced meal. You may believe dessert goes with dinner, and you can honor that with a small adjustment. Again it is a practice of giving yourself permission and doing it in a way where you will eat much less. By having dessert with dinner, you achieve the satisfaction you are looking for without eating too much. If you wait to have it later on, you will have more than you need or want and it will be a straight shot of simple carbohydrates that will spike both your blood sugars and insulin. That can lead to more cravings, hypoglycemia, insulin resistance, and more weight gain. I'll discuss more about balancing foods shortly.

As with food associations, you can change beliefs in an instant if you have immediate clarity about the behavior and if there isn't any emotional baggage attached to it. This happened for Annette when we were talking how hard it was for her to have breakfast and instead just had water. I asked her when she started doing that, and she told me at fifteen to lose weight. I then asked how well this had worked. She paused and realized it had never worked, yet she'd been doing it all her life. This was an ah-ha moment for her, and it was easy to change her belief about drinking water instead of eating in the morning when she saw the folly of it.

Georgette had her own ah-ha realization that quickly shifted her beliefs about emotional eating. She had believed once you were an emotional eater you couldn't overcome it. She was amazed as she came to recognize this was a limiting belief and not true. Maria, who never had time to eat, realized that never having time was a belief she could change into "I can make the time," and she began saying that to herself and reminding herself each week. She didn't try to change all of her behaviors at once. Instead, she made time for breakfast a few days a week and built that up to every day. And Justine, who tended to eat too much at night, recalled that growing up she was praised for taking a second helping, which filled her family and herself with pride. This was still driving her to take too much as the mother of her own family.

If you aren't so sure you can change your beliefs, you aren't alone. Clarissa was worried her beliefs were so ingrained that she wouldn't be able to change some of them. Yet by experiencing ah-ha insights, trying some new beliefs out and having strategies to support them, she discovered she could change. She said one week as she was checking in for a session that something I had said the prior week had changed her thinking, and that in turn was changing her belief and her behavior. Her new belief was, "I can have this food, I just don't have to have it now," which addressed her restrictive rebellion and frequent binges.

Perceived Pressure

Many people eat food they don't really want because they feel pressure to do so or want to please others. Tiffany didn't want to say no when offered an ice cream bar from a friend. Ginny didn't want to offend her host by leaving food on her plate. Michael couldn't say no to the pie his girlfriend made just for him. Gabriella didn't feel right eating less than those around her, and Gail felt that if her daughter had an ice cream cone then she should too. In each case, they overrode their own needs and ate beyond what they needed to meet the perceived approval or need of someone else.

I say perceived because while it may seem like pressure or judgment is coming from the other person to eat something, very often that is not the case. An assumption is being made that it's unacceptable to say no to the offer of food, stop eating before others are through or let someone eat while you don't. And that assumption is based on your own beliefs, and very often from what you were taught to do as a child. But those beliefs are outdated and very often the other person doesn't care at all whether you eat or not. If they do, it is because of their own beliefs and insecurities, which you aren't responsible for.

There are ways to be polite about your decision to eat less or not at all. You can say "No thanks, I've had enough" or "No thanks, it looks wonderful but I'm not hungry," or "I'd be happy to take it home because it so good, but I can't possibly have another bite now." Ginny gave this a try at a friend's house when she was served a plate of cookies and bowl of fruit. She didn't want anything, and she was able to say no thanks and simply have a cup of tea. She felt so much better than if she had taken care of her friend's feelings by eating to meet her needs.

Gabriella found it helpful to consider who she was eating for when she continued to eat beyond feeling satisfied. The most important person to eat for is yourself, otherwise you are giving your power away and becoming a victim to your perceptions of what others need. Consider who you are eating for and why that is when you overeat or eat when you aren't even hungry.

I am eating for _____ because _____

This belief comes from _____

The feeling I get from this is _____

What new belief will better support you now? _____

Emotional Eating

There are several types of emotional eating, where food is used as a coping mechanism for dealing with your feelings. They are restricted rebellion (representing the unmet needs and feelings of the deprived inner child), emotional repression and low self-esteem, which is a sub-set of emotional repression and worth highlighting in its own right.

Restricted Rebellion

We are taught early on in our lives to do as we are told regarding food. As children we do not have a choice about what we are served, when we will get to eat, or how much we must eat. Years ago families were more likely to eat together then they do today. Then the meal times were consistently set at specific times and children were expected to eat everything put in front of them whether they were hungry or not. Food was used as a tool for discipline by restricting food or dessert if you were bad, or giving you more of what you wanted if you were good. Some of this still happens today, but more often meals occur on the run, in the car or at the last minute and they aren't as structured or particularly healthy.

Both scenarios, however, restrict children from getting food when they are hungry, getting enough of the foods that feel good to them, or providing positive boundaries for food. In households where the parents are dieting or believe their children need to diet, further restrictions are put in place that deny children food they need or love. This isn't just prevalent today; parents have been doing this for generations.

Georgette grew up continually hungry and anxious because she couldn't ever get enough food. Her mother's dieting was a family affair and left them all in a state of deprivation. Later as she had more access to food she couldn't stop eating. She panicked if she didn't overeat for fear she might not get enough. As she got older the connection was lost and it wasn't so clear to her why she continually ate too much. Working with me she got in touch with what fullness felt like, paid attention to what she was feeling at the end of a meal, and reminded herself that she could always have more food any time she got hungry. The new pattern worked, and she was finally able to break the cycle of deprivation neediness and eat only as much as felt satisfying.

Christina's mother was bulimic and restricted her from sugar, which later became Christina's number one craving in an emotional attempt to make up for the deprivation. Jill had a different experience. Her bulimic mother was preoccupied with food yet felt helpless and terrified that eating would lead to weight gain. She wouldn't let Jill eat when she got hungry, yet made her eat when she wasn't. The craziness this created about food got passed to Jill who later struggled to recognize and honor her physical needs as an adult. She spent years denying herself sleep, water and food, following the extreme pattern set back in her childhood.

What happens at home gets compounded for children by the peer pressure they face at school to lose weight and diet. As kids and young adults experiment with restricting themselves to feel better about their appearances, they add more fuel to their enforcing inner parental voice. The more diets they try, the more restricting their beliefs about food become and the louder and more frequent the enforcer tries to control their behaviors.

If you have been restricted from food anytime in the past from either the way you were raised or from dieting, or believe you will or should be in the future, you will have an emotional reaction to this deprivation. That inner child carries emotional memories of not getting its needs met with food. At every opportunity it tries to make up for what it didn't get and to settle the associated anxiety, anger or whatever feelings are associated with the restriction of food. Not until the deprivation and feelings are acknowledged and addressed, will the child be resolved and at peace. In the meantime it will rebel against the restrictions and eat whatever it can get its hands on, no matter how much you try to control your behavior and will yourself to be good.

To resolve this rebelling behavior, have compassion for yourself. When you find yourself overeating or bingeing, be curious and gentle. Focus on what you are feeling and why.

I am feeling _____ because _____
and what else...

I am feeling _____ because _____

By acknowledging your feelings about being restricted around specific foods you are bringing them out into the open where they are no longer repressed. You are also getting a glimpse into the enforcer. Stuart was feeling a craving for potato chips because he wanted to indulge. He was also feeling guilty about the indulgence because he knew he shouldn't have them.

The next step is to look at your beliefs that the enforcer is using to bully the child. Why shouldn't you have what it is that you want?

I shouldn't _____ because _____

Who says? Is this really an appropriate restriction for you now?

This belief comes from _____

Does this belief serve you or is it holding you back from getting your needs met? _____

If it doesn't serve you, can you give yourself permission to eat the foods you want? _____

What new belief will better support you now? _____

You may find as you do this questioning that it isn't just food you've been deprived of that is driving you to overeat. You may have been restricted from specific types of meals, certain experiences, time just for you, not being taken care of, or any number of things that feel depriving to you. In turn, you may be turning to food to make up for those losses.

Emotional Repression

Emotional repression is what most associate with emotional eating. Early on we learn that expressing ourselves is not always acceptable, and we start to bury the feelings where no one can see or hear them. In the process, the feelings move below the surface and into our subconscious where they remain silently active. As other events occur that touch on these sensitivities, we may over react or have an emotional response that otherwise wouldn't occur. The more that gets buried, the more easily we become triggered. When you can't express these triggered emotions or get your needs met than food acts as a feel good substitute. Food pacifies, soothes and numbs. Chocolate in particular also temporarily makes you feel happy because it activates several "happy" neurotransmitters in the brain.

Karl found the whole idea of looking at his feelings very uncomfortable. He didn't want to mess around in them and binged just thinking about the process – that is until he actually went through it and discovered that bringing up feelings doesn't mean you have to go back and deal with past experiences. He discovered the process of feeling his emotions and having clarity stopped the emotional eating and helped him come up with strategies to meet his needs.

He had a particularly rough week of overeating once and didn't know why he had lost control. I asked him what he was feeling when he overate and when he first noticed this. As he went through the *"I was feeling... because..."* exercise with me he began to have one insight after another. He realized that an experience with a friend triggered him and that the underlying feelings were feeding fuel to the experience and being placated with comfort foods.

Tami had a similar experience when her best friend didn't show up as scheduled when they had made plans. She was new in the area and didn't have any other friends to do things with, so she did what always worked to block the pain by gorging on sugary foods and chocolate. The next day, as she sat with her hangover, she began asking herself what she was feeling and why. Here's what she wrote.

I am feeling hurt because the only friend I had blew me off.

I am feeling lonely because I don't have other friends I can call and do things with.

I am feeling anxious because I hate being alone.

I am feeling vulnerable because I don't know if I'll make more friends.

I am feeling unwanted because back in college I didn't make friends easily and felt left out.

I am feeling unlovable because my old brothers didn't include me in things.

I am feeling unworthy because I'm different from others and don't always fit in.

She realized that she was carrying a belief that she was different and perhaps unworthy of having friends, and she was feeling hurt, lonely, anxious and vulnerable. She let herself cry and wrote a lot more in her journal to let the feelings come out. She hadn't thought about trying to hang out with her brothers for years and was surprised this even came up. She had no idea it had bothered her that much, but now she could see that it did. She could also see how much she missed the friends that she had just left and got a chance to grieve over the loss, which she hadn't done in all the busyness of moving. And she realized that she needed to be more proactive to meet women in the area and make new friends.

When you are dealing with feelings that are repressed, keep asking yourself what else you are feeling and see where it leads you.

If Tami had stopped after the first two insights, she wouldn't have gotten to what was really driving her to eat. Once she released the pain and sadness and knew what it was she could do to address her current loneliness, she was less likely to have these feelings drive her behavior in the future.

I am feeling _____ because _____
and what else…

I am feeling _____ because _____
and what else…

I am feeling _____ because _____
and what else…

I am feeling _____ because _____
and what else…

I am feeling _____ because _____

As I mentioned once before, feelings about past events may surface but you don't have to get into them. If the feelings do come up, simply feel the feeling you are having in that moment, see if you have beliefs that no longer serve you, and identify what it is you need now.

I believe _____

If this belief isn't supporting you or any longer true, change it to a new belief

I now believe _____

And what needs aren't getting met that you want to address, and how will you meet them?

I need _____

I will _____

After Tami wrote about how she felt and cried, she focused on what she needed in the present moment and that was a strategy for making new friends. She felt back in control and understood what had triggered her sugar binge. She started going to local networking events and began playing tennis at a sports club, and soon she had several good friends with whom she could always rely on to do things.

Not everyone feels the need to cry or physically express their emotions; many get relief just by acknowledging and sitting with their feelings and allowing themselves to feel sad, mad, frustrated, disappointed, empty, lonely, excited, delighted or whatever else that comes up. Ginny felt overwhelmed when she was constantly surrounded by people. She had grown up an only child and was used to having time and space to herself. When she didn't get it, she was uncomfortable and didn't feel in control. It was easy to lose her bearings and turn to food, particularly when she had family visiting for extended periods of time. Once she understood the connection, she was able to get her feelings out on paper and find ways to give herself some breathing space when she had company.

Very often there are multiple feelings to process, not just one. Nicholas realized he was sad, angry and lonely, and they were inextricably linked with the death of his mother when he was a child. As he became more aware of these emotions, he observed how sensitive he was and why he was so easily triggered to overreact or turn to food. While he had dealt with his mother's early death in therapy he could see that he had more grieving and processing to do. Just allowing the feelings to come up and be visible helped.

Diane grew up in a family that didn't express emotions because it made her parents too uncomfortable. She had no frame of reference for identifying her feelings, much less a way to release them. Yet she was open to the process and felt so much better each time she got out what she was feeling. She learned that the more you push feelings down, the more they fester and eat at you. Once she got some of her feelings out, she felt freer and lighter. She immediately noticed that she was turning to food less out of emotional hunger.

Many people, and I used to be one of them, don't really know how to identify their feelings. If you haven't grown up being able to say what you feel, you may not even fully know what a feeling is, so it helps to have a list. I have put one together (in the Appendix) that is based in part on a list out of Linda Spangle's book *Life is Hard, Food is Easy*, which by the way offers good suggestions for how to express your feelings and get your needs met.

Low Self-Esteem
What we believe and feel about ourselves defines our self-esteem. It is your own self-appraisal of your worthiness, and it becomes the basis for how you judge your body, behaviors and abilities. Disordered eating, weight issues and self-esteem often go hand in hand. The worse you believe about yourself, the more likely you will bury the feelings about that with food. The heavier you get, the more ashamed you feel and will turn to food to push the feelings away.

Those that have high self-esteem have confidence in themselves, reassuring self-talk, positive self-image and enough self–respect to set healthy boundaries.

People with low self-esteem feel unworthy, undeserving and less than good enough. This is continually reinforced by their harsh inner critic that reminds them of everything that is wrong with them and what they are doing that is bad. They struggle to see they are deserving of getting their needs met, taking care of themselves or setting boundaries. Instead they are susceptible to giving their power away to others in an attempt to please them and look for reassurance of favor. The same thing happens with food. You give your power away to food when you deprive yourself of it and lose control in its presence. You also become a willing victim of food, when you eat it to satisfy someone else, use it to get your needs met, rebel against the inner critic, or deliberately sabotage your efforts by proving you are indeed bad and a failure.

I spent much of my youth and adult life with low self-esteem and believed I wasn't good enough as compared to those around me. I didn't think I was deserving of getting or having what I wanted, which led to a continual feeling of shame, denying myself of enjoyment, and feeling sorry for myself. My subconscious belief that I was unacceptable for who I was, taken on from my experiences as a child, drove my self-sabotaging choices and behaviors. Dieting and the restrictions I had to deal with because of food intolerances suited me. I was a vigilant enforcer of the rules, and the stricter the rules the more I felt deserving of them. I would clamp down even more after my restricted child had gotten the upper hand and I had overindulged on the forbidden foods. It took non-judgmental love of myself to break the cycle.

A number of my clients tell me right up front they want help building their self-esteem and feeling better about themselves. They want to be more accepting of their bodies, forgiving of their behaviors and confident of their abilities. Abigail was one of them, and she no longer wanted to feel like a victim of food. As she learned to observe her eating and drinking behaviors without judging them, she discovered that she drank or ate too much when she was trying to do what others wanted instead of focusing on her own needs.

She realized she put her needs last in an attempt to reach the pinnacle of being good enough. Yet she could never reach it because the reason she felt she had to be better was coming from her past. It was an unresolved issue with someone who would never understand her and whom she was never going to be able to please. When she began to see she was enough, she could say no to the things she didn't want to do, and she could focus on getting her own needs met. She also saw that the better she felt about herself, the more she was willing to take care of herself.

Doreen was also an overachiever, trying to win favor with the abusers of her childhood and marriage. There were times she was so depressed, she didn't feel entitled to feed herself. Other times she overate because she was disgusted with herself or didn't feel worthy of taking better care. By taking her power back with food, giving herself permission to eat forbidden foods, listening to her hunger levels and honoring them, and forgiving herself, she regained some confidence and self-respect. She reframed her belief that she had to be perfect with *good is good enough*, and she took time to acknowledge the ways in which she was doing well. It became clear to her that shame and self-criticism were driving her unhealthy relationship with food and dysfunctional eating behaviors.

Becoming Free Once You Understand Yourself

So far the discussion has been about behaviors around food, yet you may discover, as most of my clients have, that what you learn about yourself in the process will be less about food than you might think. The way you deal with food is a mirror for the way you deal with other things in your life, and your ah-has and discoveries about your beliefs, feelings and behaviors toward food will give you insights that will help you create other positive changes.

There is incredible freedom once you come to understand what has been driving your behaviors around food. No longer do you have to beat yourself up or be led by your antiquated beliefs, inner voices or repressed emotions. As you uncover these and let them go, you will likely feel relief and a renewed sense of confidence. You will also be able to focus on what you really want and need, and give yourself permission to have these and to take care of yourself in a way that feels so much better. Once you do this, you won't want to do what others want just to please them, and you will discover it really isn't selfish or rude to stand up for herself or get your needs met. Actually it is welcomed because when you aren't happy and content, most likely those around you aren't either. Everyone benefits when you respect yourself and get what you really want.

The toughest part of the process is remembering to ask yourself what you are feeling or thinking whenever you overeat, eat when you aren't hungry, or choose foods that make you feel sick. Some of my clients have an index card with the questions on them that they keep in the kitchen or carry with them. Others write them on the journal pages. You have to experiment with what works best for you. If you don't remember to ask yourself, you won't get the insights and you won't easily be able to change your behaviors.

Clarity through understanding is the second C, and it is what changes your mindset and your relationship with food and yourself. Once you have displaced the diet mindset and beliefs that kept you stuck in the see-saw of deprivation and overeating, you become free to eat the things you enjoy most and experience the pleasure and satisfaction of food.

UNDERSTAND WHAT DRIVES YOUR BEHAVIORS

What clues are you getting from your discovery journal about underlying triggers?

How would you label your inner voices, and what roles do they play?

    What triggers each of the voices, and what do they need?

What food associations are you noticing, and what other things could become new associations?

What are some beliefs you have about how, when or what you should eat?

    How can you change your beliefs so they support you better?

Who are you eating for and why do you think that is?

What rules are you carrying around that restrict you from having the foods you want when you want them?

    How can you give yourself permission now to have those foods?

    What else have you been denied that you now want to allow in your life?

If you are eating out of repressed emotions, how did it feel to get to root of what was driving you overeat?

    What works for you to release your feelings?

    How are you now going to get your needs met?

What is helping you feel more confident and better about yourself?

Choosing Healthier Options You Enjoy

You may think you know what you should eat and which foods are healthy. Yet I've found that most people equate healthy choices with dieting recommendations and just as many are still confused about simple and complex carbohydrates. It has gotten more difficult to know how to make healthy food choices, not easier.

The easiest way to make healthy choices is to understand basic nutrition, which is surprisingly simple. What complicates things are dieting restrictions, tips in magazines, a new diet or weight loss book, and the constant research findings indicating a specific food is good or not good for you. Pick any theory or belief, and no doubt someone has written about it or funded research on it, giving a thumbs up or thumbs down. The best thing to do is focus on the basics and what feels right to your body. Without this, you can't determine for yourself if someone's advice, whether an expert or not, makes sense or if it is best for you.

Understanding Basic Nutrition

Nutrition is the process through which our cells use nutrients to sustain life. Nutrients are protein, carbohydrates, fat, vitamins, minerals and water. We need all of them throughout the day to replenish our cells and support our metabolism.

Our focus here will be on carbohydrates, protein and fat – the three primary elements of food.

Carbohydrates are the main source of energy for maintaining your metabolic rate. It is also the source of fiber for digestion and glucose for brain functioning. Protein builds and repairs tissues, which is why body builders need more of it than the rest of us. It is also necessary for the replenishment of hormones and enzymes. Fat is needed for healthy skin, cell functioning and additional energy reserves. All are vital to our health, so you don't want to severely cut out or restrict any of them during the day.

Carbohydrates	Protein	Fat
Primary source of energy	Used to build & repair tissue	Part of cell membrane
Energy used by the brain	Replenishes hormones	Maintains skin & hair
Source of fiber for digestion	Supports fluid transport	Secondary source of energy

If you aren't sure which food falls into each of these categories, you are not alone. Nearly everyone has some confusion about this.

Carbohydrates are either simple or complex. Simple carbohydrates are often recognized as the "white stuff" — think pastries, bagels, white bread, baked potato, white rice, pasta and crackers. They are often made with refined or enriched flours and don't list a whole grain first in the label. Usually the amount of sugar as a percent of total carbohydrates is fairly high. You may be surprised to learn that ice cream and milk are mostly a simple carbohydrate. So too are fruit and fruit juices as well as carrots and corn because of their high sugar content. It is easy to label simple carbohydrates as bad carbohydrates, but that isn't true.

Moderate amounts of fruit, milk, chocolate, wine and many other simple carbohydrates have nutritional value. For example, fruit contains vitamins, minerals and fiber. Milk gives you calcium, vitamin D and other nutrients. Dark chocolate contains flavonoids, which have antioxidant properties. Wine also has flavonoids, and red wine in particular has other chemical properties believed to be beneficial. Even sugar has value as a simple carbohydrate, when it is used to rapidly replenish blood sugar levels after an intense aerobic activity or a hypoglycemic event. Not only that, sugar makes many foods and beverages taste more satisfying. Instead of writing off simple carbohydrates as bad foods, try enjoying them in small quantities.

Complex carbohydrates (now being called good carbohydrates) are dense with lots of fiber and very little sugar, and they are generally whole foods with minimal processing. These carbohydrates include nearly all vegetables, whole grains and beans. The good news is that many of the simple carbohydrate foods I mentioned, like pasta, breads and cereal, are now being made with 50% or more whole grains and less sugar. That means you can find more complex alternatives for simple carbohydrates you really enjoy.

Fat is either saturated or unsaturated. Saturated fats, as well as trans fats, increase cholesterol. Saturated fats primarily come from animal products, such as meats and dairy products (butter, cheese, cream). Unsaturated fats, including Omega 3 fats, help improve cholesterol and reduce heart disease. These fats primarily come from plants, like olive or flax seed oil, and from nut butters and fish. There are a few exceptions, such as coconut and palm oil, both of which are relatively high in saturated fat.

Protein is divided into lean protein and fatty protein. Lean protein choices are white meats, lean cuts of red meat, most fish and reduced-fat processed meats. Fatty protein is primarily red meats, dark poultry, and processed meats such as bacon, sausage, hot dogs, bologna and cold cuts. These are high in saturated fat. Fortunately, butchers and manufacturers are finding ways to reduce the fat and you can now find lean cuts of meat and chicken or turkey sausage and bacon.

The chart on the following page can help you quickly identify the primary categories that foods fall into. The sections with high simple carbohydrates and saturated fats have grey backgrounds to remind you that these are best eaten in moderation.

Simple carbohydrates have less nutrient value than complex carbohydrates, and they carry a high glycemic index because of their higher sugar content. This is particularly important to diabetics because the faster a carbohydrate breaks down; the faster it elevates blood sugar levels and the need for insulin. Even for those not dealing with diabetes this is important to avoid. Elevated blood sugars and the associated insulin response can lead to a roller coaster of excessively high and then low blood sugars that in turn can become Reactive Hypoglycemia, insulin resistance and then type 2 diabetes. It can also create moodiness, sugar and carbohydrate cravings, headaches and the inability to lose weight. Not only that, when insulin is high, bio-chemically you don't easily release fat.

Saturated fat is not the same as the unsaturated fat we need. Unsaturated fat gives us the essential fatty acids for our cellular health, skin, hair and energy. Saturated fat (and trans fat), on the other hand, raises blood cholesterol and puts you at greater risk for heart disease and stroke.

It does not mean you should completely avoid simple carbohydrates and saturated fats. In small quantities along with other foods they are just fine, and may make all the difference between feeling satisfied or deprived. It doesn't take much, and often less than you think, to enjoy these foods you love. If you deprive yourself and choose an alternative to be good, no doubt you will find yourself unsatisfied and trying to make up for that unmet need. It's better to have what you really want instead.

That said, many foods high in saturated fat and simple carbohydrates can be replaced with healthier options in the other food categories. For example, you can find lean cuts of beef and sausage made from chicken or turkey instead of from beef and pork. You can also now easily find yummy whole grain crackers, pasta and breads that taste just as good as those made with refined flours. If you like them just as much, you will be able to have more of the things that aren't so easily replaced.

Complex Carbohydrate	Simple Carbohydrate	Lean Protein	Fatty Protein
Whole grain breads/...	White bread/bagel/roll/cracker	Chicken breast	Chicken - dark
Whole grain pastas	Refined grain pasta	Turkey breast	Turkey - dark
Whole grain cereals	Refined grain cereals	Beef – lean cuts	Beef
Brown/wild/basmati Rice	White rice	Ham	Honey baked ham
Quinoa and other grains	Baked goods/pastry	Hamburger – lean	Hamburger
Green vegetables	Desserts	Sausage – lean	Sausage
Most other vegetables	Corn, carrots, beets, tomato	Pork	**Saturated Fat**
Most potatoes	Baked/instant potatoes	Fish	Butter
Root vegetables	Fruits	**Lean Protein &**	Margarine
Beans/soy beans/lentils	Fruit juices	**Mostly Unsaturated Fat**	Cream
	Jam/jelly	Peanut butter	Cheese
	Sugar/honey/syrup	Nuts	Whole milk
	Simple Carbohydrate & Protein (some with Saturated Fat)	Seeds	**Unsaturated Fat**
		Cottage cheese	
		Low fat cheese	Canola oil
	Milk	Low fat milk	Olive oil
	Ice cream	Soy milk	Vegetable oils
	Yogurt	Soybeans	Flax oil
		Tofu	Fish oil
		Egg	Avocados/olives
		Fish	

Protein is listed in the last two columns, but they can also be found in plant-based complex carbohydrates. You might be surprised by how much protein is in your vegetables and grains. Most plant-based foods though won't have all nine of the essential amino acids of a complete protein that animal-based products have. Beans and some vegetables and grains do have all nine, yet the quantity is typically low. For vegetarians, therefore, it is necessary to combine foods — or at least eat a combination of foods during the day — to get a full supply of all the essential amino acids that the body cannot produce itself. The rule of thumb is to either combine beans with grains, dairy or nuts or to combine grains with dairy, beans or nuts. These combinations create complete proteins.

This approach to grouping foods into their primary nutrient category is the first step to changing your relationship with food. Up until now you have probably thought about a specific food as good or bad, which has kept you caught up in the battle between the enforcer, deprived child and inner critic. The way out is to think of foods by their function and to open up the door to flexible options. Instead of looking at your plate and thinking you should or shouldn't have what's on it, think of what is there in terms of the balance of food categories and which categories are most represented. This removes the judgment since carrots, chocolate and pastry are all simple carbohydrates. And truthfully there is no bad food except for those with trans-fat, which isn't really a food but a manufactured way of stabilizing fats.

Balancing Foods for Healthy Satisfaction

Balance is the operative word for creating healthy meals and snacks. First, balance includes having a balance of carbohydrates, protein and fat that ensures you are replenishing the nutrients and energy for health throughout each day. Second, balance is eating regularly throughout the day in alignment with your hunger levels in order to maintain optimal blood sugar and metabolism levels.

The ideal and healthiest balance of foods is a combination of complex carbohydrates along with some lean protein and unsaturated fat, even at snack times. Examples are whole grain toast and peanut butter, oatmeal with low-fat milk, egg and whole grain toast with jam, spinach salad with an unsaturated fat dressing, stir fry with brown rice, whole grain pasta with a meat sauce, fruit and low-fat cheese, or hummus and whole grain crackers. Do you see that these all have protein, carbohydrates and fat and focus on the healthier types?

Additional examples are pizza, cheese and crackers, sandwiches, Paninis, cereal and milk, omelet and hash browns, spaghetti and meatballs. These are all balanced choices even though they may be high in saturated fats and simple carbohydrates. If you love these foods, then instead of depriving yourself of them see if you can find ways to make it a bit healthier. You don't have to find alternatives for every ingredient unless that is easy and satisfying for you to do.

Pizza is actually a great choice because it is inherently balanced. Many of my clients have found healthier variations in the frozen food section, on line or at a local pizza place specializing in fresh options.

Here's a way to eat a healthier pizza

- Replace the refined flour crust with a whole grain crust.
- Replace the high saturated cheese with a lower fat cheese and have a bit less of it.
- Replace the sausage and pepperoni with a leaner meat or a leaner sausage and pepperoni. There are a lot of meats being cut and processed with considerably less saturated fat.
- Replace the tomato sauce with one that has less sodium.
- Then consider adding some vegetables.

With the changes you don't lose much flavor and you have converted a high calorie and high fat, simple carbohydrate pizza into a complex carbohydrate, lean protein and lower saturated fat balanced meal. You can create healthier meals and snacks by replacing or reducing the ingredients of any recipe that has a lot of simple carbohydrates or saturated fats.

You might be pleasantly surprised by what is now available from food manufacturers if you haven't looked for alternatives lately. You can often find things that are similar to what you already eat that is just as tasty and much healthier. I often tell people to go to the grocery store and take a fresh look at what is in the aisles. There are continually new and improved products with more whole grains and healthier fats with less sugar and sodium, and most of them taste very good. Don't assume you can't have bacon, as Mandy did when I took her to the store. Assume that you can find a healthy alternative to your favorite foods and be willing to try various brands for the one that tastes best to you.

My client Ellis discovered he could create healthier variations quite easily when he started taking a look at foods differently. He was concerned he would be put on blood pressure and cholesterol medications if he didn't get his levels under control. When he came to me, he had just over a month before he had to go for blood work and a decision would be made about putting him on medication. The idea of taking pills for the rest of his life was not something he wanted to do, nor did he want to go on a restricted diet that would be hard to live with.

We discussed what he was eating during the day, and I helped him tweak his choices so he could reduce the saturated fats, sodium and simple carbohydrates without really changing what he was eating. For breakfast he ate English muffins with butter and peanut butter. I asked him to try 100 percent whole wheat English muffins with just peanut butter and see if that tasted just as good to him. He said it tasted almost the same. By making a slight shift, he was eating complex instead of simple carbohydrates and eliminated the high saturated fat in the butter. For lunch he liked roast beef sandwiches, and he discovered that he could get leaner cuts of roast beef at the deli and switch to a whole grain bread with reduced fat mayonnaise without losing the flavor he enjoyed. He started checking labels to see which products were higher in sodium and saturated fat and choosing brands that were healthier, and he reduced how much butter he was using when he cooked. He loved how little his way of eating and the flavors he enjoyed was changed, and how much better he felt. And a month later his blood pressure and cholesterol levels were down just enough to avoid the medications. He has been medication-free ever since.

Ideally you will find a way to always have fat and or protein with carbohydrates whenever you eat. If you just have carbohydrates at a sitting, say a piece of fruit or a bagel or a combination of low-fat yogurt and a banana, then chances are good that you will be hungry within two hours, low in energy and somewhat unsatisfied. Try adding in some protein and fat to reduce the high glycemia impact of the carbohydrates, slow down the digestive process and increase your nutrients and satisfaction. If you eat primarily fat and protein, such as nuts, and skip the carbohydrates then you are depleting your metabolic need for fuel and may end up eating more fat and protein than you need in a day.

The recommended guidelines for how much carbohydrate, protein and fat to eat are fairly straightforward. It is 50-55 percent of your calories as carbohydrates, 20-25 percent as protein and 25 percent as fat. It is a bit more complicated than that, however, because we measure our food in grams, and fat is twice as dense in grams per calorie than carbohydrates or fat.

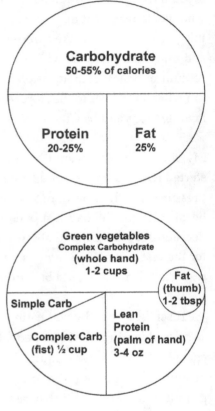

For example, if your metabolic rate is 2,000 calories a day, then you would want to strive for about 1,000 calories of carbohydrates, 500 calories of protein and another 500 for fat.

In grams this would be:

Carbohydrates: 1000 / 4.1 = 244 grams
Protein: 500 / 4.3 = 115 grams
Fat: 500 / 9.1 = 55 grams

How these food categories would look on a plate is not quite the same as the pie chart above because fat is usually in or on things and only amounts to about a tablespoon and because greens have so few calories as compared to the denser grains, beans and root vegetables. Shown here (to right) is one possible way of balancing a luncheon or evening meal. It is meant to give you some perspective as you look at the foods on your own plate.

As you can see I made room for a bit of simple carbohydrates, such as corn, fruit or a dessert, but you may instead opt for more complex carbohydrates in its place.

Balancing your foods is not an exact process of counting and measuring, although you may want to do that a few times to get an idea of portions and calories for your metabolism and hunger levels. Then I urge you to stop measuring and counting, lest you start giving the enforcer more ammunition to try and control and deprive you.

Calorie counting is the fastest way to give your power back to your inner critic and enforcer and to get pulled back into the diet mentality. Let that go and trust that the 3 Cs of consciousness, clarity and choices will guide you more effectively. Like those who are naturally thin and healthy or the French women who don't get fat, focus on your hunger levels and reaching satisfaction.

After working together for about a month, Michael began writing down his foods in the discovery journal to see how well his choices were balanced. For the most part, he had already begun to balance things because it felt better to him, but seeing it and then describing how each meal was or wasn't balanced with me helped him get a better understanding and more ideas for what would work better.

On the day shown below, you can see he was consistently eating when he got hungry and stopping when he was satisfied. This was now fairly normal for him, and when he got too hungry he knew it and had something ready to eat to address it.

Name: Michael	Date: 5/14	M T W TH F Sa Su													
						Hunger Scale								
Time	Food	Quantity	0	1	2	3	4	5	6	7	8	9	10	Mood - Thoughts - Feelings
7:15	Corn flakes Milk Orange juice	1 cup 1/2 cup 8 oz			X				X					Enjoyed this, but not sure it is all that balanced
10:20	Kashi bar Banana	1 1		X						X				Wow, I was so hungry by 10 and as soon as I got out of my meeting I went right for my stash of bars. Thank God I knew I had these or I would have eaten several donuts. Having a good day and the meeting went well
1:00	Turkey rollup on ww wrap mayo, vegetables Small bag of potato chips	1 1			X					X				Out with the team and this was perfect
4:15	Apple Mixed nuts	1 1/4 cup			X					X				Busy, but I did notice getting hungry and had the apple from lunch
7:30	Grilled chicken breast Grilled corn on the cob Grilled zucchini/squash Brownie	1 1 1/2 cup 1			X					X				Beautiful evening to grill and enjoy some spring weather Feeling good and productive Very satisfying meal and had one of my favorite kind of brownies

What he noticed as we walked through this day was how unbalanced breakfast was. He was right. Cornflakes, milk and orange juice are all primarily simple carbohydrates, which isn't the best way to start the day. There was some protein in the milk, but not enough to offset the carbohydrates. So it isn't surprising he was really hungry a few hours later, particularly since he didn't quite have enough to begin with to even be satisfied. Then he had a banana, which is another simple carbohydrate, with his Kashi bar that is fairly well balanced, so this was a bit weighted to carbohydrates yet balanced all the same. As importantly he refueled his energy and metabolism.

He was then able to go another few hours comfortably and be hungry at lunch time. He had a well balanced lunch that included a turkey rollup and a handful of chips, which was fine because only the chips had saturated fat and it was in moderation. It also satisfied him. About three hours later he had some nuts and an apple, which is a nice balance of protein and fat in the nuts and carbohydrates from the apple. And three hours after that he enjoyed another healthy meal that balanced lean protein (chicken breast), complex carbohydrates (zucchini and squash), simple carbohydrate (corn) and fat (in all the foods) and a small dessert to satisfy his nighttime sweet tooth. I noticed he was eating every few hours, honoring his hunger levels and satisfying his needs. He also knew when something wasn't balanced and got feedback from his body when he didn't eat enough at a previous meal.

If the enforcer had its way, Michael would have had less simple carbohydrates and saturated fats that day, but it has learned that being in balance in combining foods and eating regularly throughout the day is more important than perfection. Michael made huge strides in choosing healthier foods on a regular basis, getting control of his portions, seldom overeating and firing up his metabolism. He was also happier, more energized and getting excited about cooking and eating to be satisfied.

When you are ready to start writing down your foods, focus on the balance of nutrients and not on the specific foods. Look at each meal and see in what way it is or isn't balanced from a neutral point of view. This isn't the place for your inner critic to judge you. This is a learning process that takes some time to get under your belt, and you only learn by evaluating your choices against the nutrient categories and observing how the different combinations affect you physically. This is a discovery process that you can use to be creative.

Joellen told me that she really liked the process and was experimenting to see what she could balance with foods she loved to eat. Barbara found that eating in balance kept her from getting too hungry or being obsessed with food. Daphne learned she craved sugar from not being satisfied when she ate and having too many simple carbohydrates in her meals. She got creative in her attempt to better balance her meals and reconnected with her love for whole foods. As she paid more attention to her hunger, she noticed a greater interest in the taste of foods and rediscovered how much she loved putting goat cheese and tomato on a WASA cracker. She also loved whole grain calzones with low saturated fat cheese. She learned that satisfaction for her was in the flavor and consistency, and she began to feel much better eating this way.

Most of my clients discover that balanced eating and healthier food choices taste much better than what they were eating before. Many also start to find they like vegetables, after avoiding them for years, and they even like to cook. Annette found she started getting hungry for greens and was eating a lot more of them by choice within five weeks. Ginny and Monica both found they really wanted more vegetables and it wasn't that hard to add them into their meals. Patricia was having fun with her salads and exploring to see which types of vegetables she might like to add. Tiffany knew she loved vegetables and healthier foods but just didn't eat them. She was reminded how much she really enjoyed them once she started eating them again.

Clarissa never liked how much work it was to cook, much less prepare vegetables, and she discovered it wasn't as bad as she thought. Stuart grew up with canned vegetables and hated them, but he started to enjoy the taste of fresh vegetables because it was now a choice and not forced on him. He even started cooking and had a lot of fun going to the store and getting more involved in what was being put on his plate. Karl started calling himself a stir fry master after coming up with a signature dish that included lots of vegetables, foods he had avoided eating for years. As you can see, it can be fun and rewarding to reintroduce foods you once thought you didn't like or were too much work to prepare.

I hope you are learning that with balanced eating you have lots of options, not less. Instead of looking at food choices as a list of what you should or shouldn't have, you can look at them as a way to create healthier meals and snacks you really enjoy in unlimited combinations. In time you will naturally and automatically look at the foods you are putting on your plate or in your bowl in terms of balancing complex carbohydrates, lean proteins and unsaturated fats and perhaps a bit of the other for greater satisfaction.

Making Room for Restricted Foods

You may rationally agree that balanced eating makes sense, and you may have already seen changes in your eating habits from using the techniques and suggestions so far in this book. Yet there may be some foods you just don't think you can have around without losing control or bingeing, and it may even feel scary to have those foods in the house. This is understandable if your restricted inner child has been unable to stop eating them in the past. The more forbidden the food is or the more the child loves that food, the more out of control you may feel.

I addressed this earlier when I talked about Subconscious Beliefs and Nicholas' approach to junk food , yet so many people struggle with the idea of allowing *bad* foods as a healthy choice that I want to address it again more specifically.

If there is a food you want such as ice cream, you can calm both of your inner voices by first giving yourself permission to have it and reminding yourself that when you want more there is an easy way to get it (satisfying the child) and secondly by determining how you can limit the quantity, make it part of a balanced meal or snack, and honor your hunger levels (thus satisfying the enforcer). It is best to start trying this after you've become familiar with fullness and are more conscious of your hunger levels, so you are paying attention to when you've had more than you really want. It is also best to plan these foods into your balanced meal or snack, so you aren't eating them separately. This avoids mindless eating and driving up your blood sugars.

Limiting the quantity may take some strategizing. Consider ways you can purchase a single serving or packaged serving sizes, and be sure it isn't too difficult to get more if you really want it. This is important because a child needs to know it won't be deprived in the future, whether that future is an hour, day, week or month later. Clarissa loved Milano cookies and would eat a whole box at a sitting, so it scared her to buy them. We talked about ways she could get them in smaller quantities, and she discovered they were sold in sealed packs of four in a box. She was willing to give this a try, and was thrilled to tell me that it worked. She was able to have just one package of four as part of her dinner, and she didn't even want them every night.

This strategy worked well until she ran out of them and tried another type of cookie that didn't come in separate little packages. She wasn't prepared for that and ate them all, which frightened her. She wondered if she would also go back to eating the whole package of Milano cookies the next time she got them. She didn't. She then realized the problem was that she didn't have a strategy for bringing home a different type of cookie, and that when dealing with forbidden foods she needed to plan and prepare for bringing them into the house. She began giving herself permission to bring other types of foods into the house, developing strategies, making sure she told herself she could have it any time and planning them into her balanced meals. This worked, and she found she could even handle surprises like the time her mother came by with donuts. She only had two and didn't want the rest that were left behind and tossed them out. This was a first and a confidence booster. The more she gave herself permission, the less she felt the need to over indulge or overeat. If she did, she looked into what she was thinking and feeling. Often she found the issue didn't have to do with the food but with other things going on in her life.

Remember Maggie who drank Pepsi throughout the day. She learned the same thing. It was having permission to continue drinking Pepsi while coming up with strategies for having less and looking at the underlying issues that helped her cut back dramatically. Many of my clients have succeeded in breaking their *bad food* mentality. Anita, who loved to eat cheese puffs while on road trips, brought smaller portions with her and felt good about it. Tiffany succeeded with the three-bite rule, where she allowed herself three bites of any dessert she wanted and was able to stop at that. Bethany tried having a small piece of dark chocolate with dinner and found she didn't want a big dessert later on. Gabriella did the same with a couple of ginger snaps. Irene discovered that if she wanted to bake cookies she did just fine if she ate a couple as part of a balanced snack or meal. And Barbara allowed herself to thoroughly enjoy a brownie, realizing "this is normal."

The same thing works for those foods you get just once a year, like Girl Scout cookies. It is much harder to stop eating if you know for sure you won't see the food again for a very long time, or if you think others will be in a race with you to get as many as they can before they are all gone. Is this what happens at your house? The good thing is you have hindsight. You do know what happens and which cookies you and others love most, so you can plan accordingly. One idea is to buy even more boxes and freeze them, so you know there is plenty more to last you for months to come. Another idea is to give each person their own *unlimited* quantity that has their name on them. One of my clients decided she would get enough of her favorite cookies so she knew she could have two every single week for a year and then she'd be able to get more.

You can develop strategies for any foods or beverages that come around just once a year, including Easter and Halloween candy, eggnog, birthday cake, Thanksgiving dinner, and other holiday meals. The best thing about most of these occasions is you really can get the items any time you want. You don't have to wait until these holidays come around to satisfy your needs. Go get a little bit at any time you want and take back control of the foods that have had so much power over you. Once you do this, you might even find you don't want these foods as you thought.

This process of reincorporating once-restricted foods doesn't happen over night and may be easier with some foods than others. Give yourself permission to try different strategies, over indulge and throw out foods when you get scared. This isn't a linear process of getting from point A to point B. There will be ups and downs, and once you get to the point of being in control most of the time you may still occasionally overdo it. Let it be and move on. As Barbara once said to me, "It's amazing, every time I don't eat a healthy meal, I gravitate back to healthy options and I don't binge. I'm no longer out of control because I don't beat myself up about it."

Planning and Preparation

One of the greatest obstacles to making healthier choices and balancing meals is the planning and preparation involved. You can be aware you are getting hungry, but if you don't have access to food you can't honor that hunger and may find yourself grabbing anything you can get your hands on or overeating when you finally do sit down to a meal.

Having Food for When You Get Hungry

Christina had gone shopping at the mall and didn't think about whether she'd get hungry. But the longer she shopped the hungrier she became. When she got back to her car, she was starving and found herself gobbling down cupcakes meant for a preschool class. Gabriella had a tendency of working as long as she could before going for lunch or leaving at night, and by the time she ate lunch or dinner she was so hungry she couldn't stop eating until she was over full. Simone also had a hard time stopping to eat during the day and made up for it by overeating at night. Daphne ate when and what was convenient during the day and seldom ate for hunger or satisfaction, so she tended to crave sugar and overeat when she did finally sit down at night.

With a little 20/20 hindsight and planning, all of them found ways to eat something balanced at the point they got hungry by recognizing they needed to think ahead. Just as with a child going off to school or an outing for the day, you want to plan and prepare the meals, snacks and beverages you need while you are working, going out or taking care of your family. You wouldn't let a child go off without doing that, so why let this happen to you.

The easiest thing to have with you in the car, out shopping, at your desk or traveling is a breakfast or meal replacement bar. Some call them generically Power bars, but many sports power bars are too heavily loaded with protein, which is not well balanced and caters to people who are weight lifting. Ideally you want a bar that is 50 percent carbohydrates, 25 percent protein and 25 percent fat — just as I talked about earlier in the section on nutrition. You also want to look for bars with less than 100 mg of sodium and under 15 grams of sugar (or sugar that is less than 40 percent of the total carbohydrates). Even better is finding a bar closer to 5 grams of sugar. In addition the more grams of fiber it has, the more complex carbohydrates are in it.

Kashi granola bars are the only ones I've seen with sugar close to 5 grams, yet the protein isn't very high. In contrast the Kashi GoLean chewy bars have a better balance of carbohydrates, protein and fat but the sugar is 31 grams (nearly 70 percent of the total carbohydrates). Personally I would err toward higher complex carbohydrates and less sugar than I would a bar with more protein and high sugar. Most of us, with the exception of vegetarians, get enough protein during the day and more than enough simple carbohydrates. Their GoLean crunchy bars are actually the most balanced and have an acceptable (but still high) level of sugar at 13 grams (48 percent of the total carbohydrates). Each bar has about the same amount of fat at around 5 grams.

This shows you that you need to look at the label and compare one bar to another. There is no one best brand, although Kashi comes close because of its whole grains and use of more natural ingredients, and you may like certain types better than others. If you are eating something else with a bar, also consider how that adds into the balance equation. If you are pairing it with fruit, go for the bar with the lowest sugar. If you are having it with nuts or cheese, go for one with the lowest fat and protein.

Food bars are not the only on-the-go option. You can bring soy nuts (a great balance all on its own), whole grain crackers with peanut butter, fruit and low fat cheese, trail mix of nuts and dried fruits, cereal you can eat plain, roll ups, sandwiches, a cup of soup, or many other combinations of balanced foods that can be easy to package up and carry with you. Check out new items at the grocery store or a deli for ideas. Then always have food with you. I always carry a food bar in my purse and car just in case I need a snack in a pinch. There have been countless times I was glad I did. I also frequently have water with me. Again, you never know when you need it.

If you are like Stuart, Carmen or Kelley, you are in your car so much you need more than a snack. You need on-the-go meals you can eat while driving. Stuart drove a lot to visit with clients, Carmen had a long drive to get to her class, and Kelley was shuffling kids half her day. One answer is a cooler filled with easy to eat foods. Another is having something that goes into a thermos. And a third is having places along the way you know makes healthy foods that can easily be eaten in the car without lots of utensils and napkins. More places are opening all the time with take-out healthy foods and many grocery stores are trying to fit this need as well. Take another look in your area if you haven't looked or asked around recently.

Planning and Preparing Meals

Being prepared is also important when you are at home. Many of my clients tell me they aren't successful in eating healthier foods in balance because they haven't stocked their kitchen to do that. As Tami said once, "I don't have the right food in the house, so when I have the urge to eat I don't have better choices available and just grab whatever is there." She felt she needed a better way to plan for her meals so this wouldn't keep happening. For her, she found it helped to think in terms of being prepared for each type of meal so she knew what worked for breakfast, lunch and dinner, and then to plan for what she needed based on her plans that week for being home, at work or having dinner with her boyfriend.

Not everyone finds it easy to do meal planning or shopping, much less cooking. The majority of my clients are not comfortable cooking, and most of them are women. I didn't learn to cook until my mid forties, so this was validating for me. Nonetheless, if you don't cook or don't enjoy it, then meal planning and shopping can be challenging. The easiest thing is to find healthier balanced foods that are already prepared or nearly prepared at the grocery store or a specialty shop. Christina found a place that pre-packaged all the ingredients for an entrée with specific instructions on how to cook it at home. She loved that the work of planning and preparing was done for her, there were lots of entrees to pick from, and it was so simple to cook a home-cooked meal for her family. Karl discovered fajitas, pre-made brown rice and a stir fry Pad Thai at Trader Joes that he called the wonder meal. You can also see if you have a local deli, grocery store or business that does healthy home-cooked meals to go.

Another option is to hire a personal chef, which is often more affordable than you may think and ask them to prepare meals for the week or specific days. This is actually a great way to get foods made to your tastes or needs, and most chefs now use fresh, organic and healthy ingredients. You can usually find one in your local area. Try personalchefsnetwork.com, pchefnet.com, personalchefsearch.com or hireachef.com to find one in your vicinity.

Gail liked to cook and learned that planning made all the difference as to whether she ate a well balanced meal or grabbed lots of simple carbohydrates. If she didn't make time to plan meals for the week, make a list and then shop and cook on Sundays, she would end up eating the simplest things she could find in her cabinets and refrigerator and these were seldom healthy choices. She loved healthy, balanced foods but they took time to prepare and if she didn't get that time on the weekends she was in a jam during the week. She was just too busy in her professional life, which often included evening events, to shop and cook.

Sharon felt similarly. When her days were too full, she didn't plan for the evenings and found this became an excuse to eat anything. But she understood that she could be more mindful and plan ahead, and that by making a few changes in her schedule she would be able to have foods at home that were easy to prepare. Michael discovered that he did much better when he put it on his schedule to stop at the grocery store after work and pick up a few things that he could easily throw on the grill. He would get enough for a few days and cook it all so that he could eat leftovers the following evenings. The best part was he got to perfect his grilling skills and had fun with new recipes.

Preparing Quick Balanced Foods

Anita wanted help with specific meal planning. She was just throwing foods together and eating whatever was easiest to prepare. Vegetables she told me were too much work so she didn't make them very often. I hear that a lot. I also hear how few vegetables people really like to eat because they find them boring. I have an answer for that so they are much easier to prepare and are more enjoyable. First try to find vegetables that have been pre-cleaned and partially prepared, so that you have less work when you get home. Be aware though that the more cut up the vegetables the less nutritious and fresh they tend to be, with the exception of frozen vegetables, so look for vegetables that are minimally pre-cut or prepared. For example green beans that are bagged and just have the ends clipped, broccoli that has had the stem cut off, butternut squash that has the outer skin removed.

Now I'll share a couple of techniques to make vegetables quickly and easily that I use. If you like roasted vegetables, you can line a sheet pan with tinfoil, spray it with olive oil (using Pam or one of your own sprayers), fill the pan with a layer of vegetables, such as broccoli tops, cauliflower pieces, cut carrot, green beans, asparagus, slices of egg plant or summer squash, or practically any vegetable that you like. Spray again with olive oil and sprinkle with a mix of salt (I use kosher salt) and an herb such as thyme. Bake at 375 for 15 minutes or longer, until the vegetables start to burn a bit. This is very simple and delicious. Of course you can also do this with a metal "basket" on the grill.

Another idea is steam your vegetables with a steamer machine that you can find in most kitchen stores or a steamer basket that sits in a pot filled with water just up to the bottom of the basket. Avoid over cooking the vegetables so they remain firm and then drizzle a bit of vinaigrette or salad dressing on top. You don't need much, and since dressings are usually made with unsaturated fat it creates a good balance to your meal. Balsamic vinaigrette goes well with asparagus and Brussels sprouts. A lemony dressing goes well on green beans and broccoli, and a champagne vinegar works well on Swiss chard. Try experimenting with different types of dressings on your favorite vegetables. You may find some great combinations that will change your whole perspective on vegetables.

As with vegetables, fish and lean meats can be cooked easily and quickly with a touch of salt and pepper or a spice mix rub on the grill, in a grill pan or under the broiler and then lightly topped with a sauce from the store. Of course, you may have your own recipes and ideas. Some people try to have a half dozen balanced meal ideas that can be made with different ingredients, such as a stir fry, whole grain pasta dish, Cobb salad, hearty soup or pizza they can quickly put together during the week or have put away in containers in the freezer.

It isn't just meals that require some planning and preparation, it helps to think of what you like that is balanced and satisfying for snacks, so you have the ingredients on hand. Ginny found that multigrain WASA toast with tomatoes and a good cheese really satisfied her as a snack and as a lunch. Nicholas discovered soy nuts and had a stash of these at his desk at work and in his car. Kelley loved fruit and pared them with either peanut butter or cottage cheese. Gabriella likes rice cakes and cottage cheese, which is also one of my favorites. I also like hummus and rice crackers. All of these ideas are a balance of protein, carbohydrates and fat. Try to think of things you would like that are balanced and easy to get when you need a snack. It is also helpful to have food bars around, as discussed earlier, just in case you don't have anything else or because you really like them.

Making Mindful Choices before Getting Hungry
Sometimes the issue isn't preparing or planning what food to have with you or to make for meals. It may instead be the awareness that if you don't eat something ahead of time, you may get too hungry when you finally do eat or when you are surrounded by food at a party. As you now know if you get too hungry, you won't be in control of what or how much you eat. This can be easily avoided with some awareness and planning.

If you know you are going to eat dinner or go out to a function around 6 pm and you ate a good lunch at 1 pm, you will likely get a bit hungry around 4 or 5 pm. It might seem best to hold off eating and wait, but actually it serves you better to have a little something ahead of time so you can stay in control. This strategy helped Gabriella, who used to work right up until the point she needed to make dinner and would then nibble on things as she cooked or would cook things that were fast but not that healthy to deal with her ravenous hunger. She never noticed it at her desk, but as soon as she got to the kitchen her hunger took over. She decided to try keeping some crackers and peanut or a food bar at her desk and would have just enough to move her hunger from a 2 to a 3 or 4 as she headed upstairs to the kitchen. Then she would feel more relaxed and focused on making a balanced meal. She also found she didn't overeat as much of the meal when she did this. Justine had the same experience and began to plan late afternoon snacks into her routine, which helped her cook a healthier meal and stay mindful as she ate it with her family.

Monica found eating ahead of time useful when going to a party where there would be lots of appetizers and drinks. She was worried she would over indulge at the event and wondered what the best strategy was for this, so we discussed her options. The one that worked well for her was to eat a balanced snack ahead of time that would bring her hunger levels to about a 5. This way she could finish her eating at the party and deliberately choose five or six appetizers that looked the best with a glass of wine. Having a strategy before she went made all the difference. She enjoyed herself and had no interest in having anything more.

Penny also created strategies for when she knew she'd be tempted to overindulge, and one of these times was an annual tradition of making holiday cookies with her girlfriends. They loved spending a day making and decorating dozens of different types of cookies, although Penny confessed she always felt sick afterward from sampling each type and licking the bowls. I suggested she include a balanced meal or snack into the day and pick out a few cookies that looked the very best to her so she could fully enjoy them and the experience with her friends. She excitedly told me on our next call how well this worked. They all benefited from eating a balanced lunch along with their favorite cookies and had a great time without over doing it.

Setting Aside Time to Eat

It seems fewer people are taking time to sit down to breakfast, lunch and dinner. It is becoming a rarity for families to sit down together during the week, and more people are simply skipping meals altogether as they grab things on the go or snack throughout the day as time allows. Choices made haphazardly, on the go and out of convenience are seldom balanced, healthy or mindful. Food becomes an afterthought and wolfed down without awareness for how it feels or how much is eaten under these circumstances.

Daphne works from home, and she often feels like she is constantly running behind. She realized that when she plans her day and sits down to eat breakfast and lunch that she eats healthier, feels better and things run more smoothly. She also determined that she needed healthy food options that were quick and easy to prepare at these times, and she found them once she had a chance to focus on it and make a plan to stock them for herself. In the process, she was a better role model for her daughters by taking just as good care of herself as she took care of them.

Maria's businesses across multiple cities had her living out of three locations each week, which meant lots of travel and little time for her needs. She too needed quick and easy meals that she could sit down to three times a day. Her changing locations had been so challenging that she had skipped breakfast and lunch for years, and she knew this was having an impact on her health. She figured out what she wanted for balanced breakfast foods that she could stock at each location and picked oatmeal, cereal and food bars. She also looked for places in each area that offered healthier choices where she could go for lunch or get as take out for dinner. When she ate a good meal in the morning and midday, she seldom overate at night and she felt better and had more stamina.

Enjoying the Foods You Love

When people find out what I do for a living, the first thing they usually ask me is what I think they should eat. My answer is pick foods you love to eat for breakfast, lunch, dinner and snacks and find healthier ways of having them so you physically feel good and satisfied. As you can imagine, this isn't the answer they were expecting or hoping for. Most people are looking for the latest and greatest food rules to follow, yet as you now understand this never works or certainly not for long.

The answer is the third C of having free choice without feeling deprived or in need of perfection. Isn't it interesting, this is the opposite of what we've been told most of our lives by those we trust and by the establishments we look to for answers? Yet it is now becoming clear that dieting does not work and the restrictions in calories and choice are fueling obesity, dysfunctional eating and chronic diseases.

When you eat what you enjoy without having to drastically change your lifestyle and choices, it is much easier to eat less, gravitate toward healthier options and stick with your new behaviors. The objective isn't to follow someone else's rules for what you should eat but to tweak what you want to eat so it is healthier and more satisfying. We are meant to enjoy our food and as you experiment with your own choices I hope you find greater pleasure before, during and after you eat. Once you do, you will likely feel more relaxed, confident and in control around food.

CHOOSE HEALTHIER FOODS YOU ENJOY

What do you notice about the way your meals and snacks are balanced?

How could they be more balanced?

How could you bring a forbidden food into the house in a way that you would feel more in control?

What have you learned works best when you have foods around that feels forbidden?

What would work best for you to plan and prepare healthy foods at home?

What kind of balanced snacks can you easily have with you in case you get hungry?

What strategies do you think would work to minimize becoming ravenous before a meal or party?

If you don't take time out to eat, how could you set aside time for this on a more regular basis?

Creating Strategies for Challenging Moments

Those times when you find yourself overeating, skipping meals, eating for no reason or choosing to eat something that isn't balanced or healthy are opportunities for insight and more discoveries about yourself and possible strategies that will help you in the future. Be curious about what it is about the event that triggered your behavior and brainstorm ways you can address things differently. And if you have an event coming up that you know has been problematic in the past, then strategize ahead of time.

Most food experiences repeat themselves, so you can try different things to see what helps you manage them differently and become more familiar with what is triggering your responses. If you are overeating, is it because you aren't getting enough during the day, you have been restricted, the enforcer is trying to control you, there are food associations, or you are using food to cope? Based on what you think the issue is, what strategies can you use the next time this happens so you have more choice and control?

Bethany, as I mentioned earlier, often ate her entire sandwich at her lunch break even though it was too much, thinking that she'd be hungry later if she didn't finish it. She knew what always happened next. She would feel sick and wish she hadn't eaten so much. When she really looked at what she was doing, she knew that the issue was her belief and that half would be ample. If she did get hungry later on it would still be there, since she also knew that no one would take it or tell her she couldn't eat it at another break.

She could also see a similar pattern in the morning with cereal. She'd fill the bowl and think it looked like a lot, but once it was filled she'd eat it all and then feel overly full. By observing this from a place of neutrality, she realized she could always start with less and add more if she didn't get enough. Looking at the two scenarios that kept recurring, it became clear there was an underlying belief that food might not be available when she needed it, and she was able to shift that belief into "there would be food whenever she got hungry."

Michael discovered that when he was sick, in pain or aggravated, he reached for junk food to feel better. He would stop paying attention to his hunger levels and lost interest in trying to balance his foods. He wanted comfort and a distraction. He didn't even care if he ate healthy foods or not because the child in him was angry he was sick and unable to get to work. His new strategy for times like this was to give himself permission to eat comfort foods and to ask his girlfriend to make healthy balanced meals for him to eat in the evenings.

Patricia didn't have a lot of energy during the day and constantly overate at dinner. She had a habit of skipping meals and was open to listening to her body to change that. She began paying more attention throughout the day to her hunger and experimenting with various types of balanced breakfasts in the morning. She was amazed how well it made her feel and the amount of energy she had with this strategy.

Belinda always stopped at McDonald's for an EggMcMuffin on the days she had to commute to work. She knew this wasn't the best choice for her, but she didn't have much time in the morning to eat breakfast before she got in the car and she needed to grab something that was fast and easy when she got to work. As she considered what else could work, she decided that the problem was a lack of planning and preparation at home. She didn't have anything she could grab on the way out the door that was appealing and balanced. Her strategy was to make some extra time and prepare her own version of an EggMcMuffin at home that was healthier or have some other breakfast options she liked that she could grab easily. She also gave herself permission to stop at McDonalds periodically if she had a crazy morning or just wanted to taste the real thing, since she really loved their EggMcMuffins.

Gabriella often ate too much when she went out to eat, and her strategy was to challenge herself to bring half of her meal home so she could enjoy the rest the next day. She loved to compete with herself and this became a game she enjoyed winning. Ginny had the same strategy to eat just half the meal when her daughter cooked because she loved her daughter's cooking and often overdid it. She enjoyed having the wonderful meal again for lunch.

Carmen discovered if she stayed downstairs after dinner she always grazed on what was leftover from the meal. She decided instead that her new routine in the evenings would be to go upstairs right after dinner where she could happily read or do other things to wind down for the evening.

Clarissa tended to binge on Sunday evenings and just couldn't stop eating the candy, cookies or desserts. She came to understand that she didn't want the weekends to end or the fun to stop. She dreaded the school and work week, particularly if she hadn't had enough time to do the things she enjoyed or had enough time just for her. She was a mother and struggled with her need for time just for herself to get replenished. Her strategy was to find a few things she thought would be fun to do on her own that took varying amounts of time, some of which she could do during the week in just fifteen minutes or on weekends for longer periods. Her husband was very willing to support her and to watch the kids while she spent part of a Saturday or Sunday off on her own.

Ruth knew that every Thanksgiving she would overeat to the point of being sick when visiting her son and daughter-in-law, and it started when she arrived at their place around noon. All over the house were dishes of nuts, candy, cookies, and snack foods that she would mindlessly eat with her glass of wine as they visited for a few hours before going over to the restaurant for the traditional buffet dinner. Already having eaten enough, she would then fill up her plate at the buffet and after finishing that would try several of the desserts. She could barely get out of her chair when they got up to go. She didn't want to repeat this again and worked with me to develop a strategy. It helped that she knew what to expect.

The strategy that worked for her was to eat a balanced breakfast earlier in the day and a small balanced luncheon before heading over to her son's place. She would then scan the dishes around the house to see which things most appealed to her and would select just a couple of things that would round out her lunch and be satisfying. Then when they went to dinner, she would be nearly hungry again. At the buffet she would again scan everything and decide which things she loved the most and what would be most balanced and fill her plate with half of what she normally would. If she still felt the need for more food she could go back for more. She would also leave room for one or two small helpings of dessert that she loved the most and end the meal without becoming full. It worked. She was ecstatic when she called me after she got back. It was the first time she hadn't gorged herself and she didn't feel like she'd missed out on anything.

These examples hopefully give you an idea for how you can create your own strategies when you know certain situations are going to come up you find challenging. Another tool that helps is using the discovery journal. Even if you haven't written things down in a while, you can always journal again for a few days to see what is happening or to write down what you recall happening after a situation that left you feeling poorly and out of control. Then consider the root of the issue and if you can do things differently. You may be surprised how easily you expand your options and find strategies that work beautifully for you.

Coaching Questions to
CREATE STRATEGIES FOR CHALLENGES

What situations keep recurring that you finding challenging to control, and what do you think is making them challenging?

Do you notice any beliefs that are driving your current behaviors at these times?

What are some things you could do differently to make healthier choices and honor your hunger levels?

What do you notice when you try out your ideas?

Keeping Yourself on Track

Like anything new, it isn't always easy to stick with a change in the way you eat or to remain conscious of your hunger levels after the first few weeks of doing it, even if you do start noticing how good it feels. It helps to have accountability and support for a few months and perhaps on a monthly basis after you begin to naturally apply the three Cs of consciousness, clarity and choice.

As with being more active, give yourself permission to have days when you don't eat in balance or overeat and let it be. Roll with it, and you will gravitate back to healthier behaviors, as Barbara observed, because you won't have initiated the enforcer-child deprivation battle. If you let the enforcer get the upper hand and feel you've blown it, you may find yourself spinning out of control. You aren't perfect, and you don't have to be to succeed. Success is having more days when you are paying attention, honoring your hunger, respecting your fullness, having insights that help you create strategies, and making balanced choices. As soon as you have to be perfect, you will have more days of rebellion and resistance. Good is good enough, and it is what will help you remain consistent to increase your metabolism and reach your goals.

Checking in With Yourself

In the first few months, I do recommend you use your discovery journal daily. This is what will keep you conscious and give you clues to the underlying drivers. You may not always remember to do it, and that's okay. But the more often you do each week, the more you will learn what the real challenges are for you and what your patterns are. It is an eye-opening process that will make it easier for you to change your behaviors than anything else.

How you keep a journal is up to you, as I said earlier. You may want to have a sheet for the week instead of for a day. You may want to keep a little notebook that you carry with you wherever you go. You may want to experiment with various formats. How you do it is less important than doing it. Some of my clients find they do it in their head without the forms if they use the forms at least once a week. Again do what works for you.

If you notice you are eating for reasons other than hunger, then ask yourself what you are feeling or thinking and why. This is what really matters. Some of my clients keep an index card with the questions about feelings and beliefs in their kitchen or with their journal so they can easily be reminded of them. It helps to have a place to write down what comes up somewhere and to then brainstorm ideas for strategies.

At the end of each week, check in to see how the week went, what you observed and learned, and then to create strategies that will help you in the future. You don't need a coach. You could become accountable with a trusted friend or family member. It might even work well if you are both doing engaged in this process. Have the other person ask you what went well, what you learned, what didn't go so well, and what might help you address a similar situation in the future. Another person helps you be accountable and can support you by listening and reflecting back what they heard as you process your insights and strategies.

Weekly Check-in Process

1) Look at what went well and what you are proud of. What can you learn from these positive experiences that you want to remember and keep doing?

2) Notice how you feel physically and mentally by the changes you've made the past week.

3) Notice what didn't go as well without any judgment.

4) Also notice if there are patterns in your behaviors around food, which could give you more understanding of what is driving your behaviors.

5) Ask yourself, if you haven't already, what are you thinking or feeling and why. Then consider your beliefs, ways to release any buried emotions, and how to get your needs met without turning to food.

6) Come up with new strategies to support you when facing similar situations in the future.

7) Now think if there are any other insights or lessons learned from the past week.

8) Ask yourself some of the coaching questions that are in this section.

9) If it is appropriate to set a goal, such as look for a new snack recipe or find a healthier alternative to something you enjoy eating, then set a goal that is realistic and achievable.

If you do this without a trained coach, be sure there is an understanding with your friend or family member that you are not to be judged or told what to do under any circumstances. Only you know what is best for you and what choices best serve you. If they start suggesting what would be better or feel strongly about what the right answer should be, stop the process. They aren't helping you. It only works if you are treated as your own authority and capable of making good choices. If they offer any suggestions at all, they need to be aware that you are not obliged nor should feel any pressure to use them. This can be tricky, and it may work better in a group setting where the agreements for neutrality are more likely to be honored.

Remembering Why You Care

A change of any kind takes time and is subject to the pull of former habits, beliefs and self-talk that may sometimes seem easier to fall back on. It will help you to remind yourself why you care about making this healthy lifestyle change and to keep using the tools and asking the questions.

If you do lose touch with how your body feels when you overeat or choose unhealthy foods, practice paying attention again and you will remember why you don't like it. Feeling full isn't pleasant, and neither is feeling sick from eating lots of simple carbohydrates and saturated fats. This will help you remember why eating in alignment with your physical hunger and choosing foods that are balanced and healthier is important to you.

Celebrating Your Healthier Eating Successes

It is a great feeling to be in control around food and to feel confident in your food choices. You become free to enjoy foods once denied you and to feel normal. For many people this alone is a celebration of what they have achieved. For others they celebrate by eating out at their favorite restaurants knowing they can do that again and again because they have strategies in place and don't fear being restricted. And I've had clients celebrate by rethinking their food budget and spending more on fresh, organic ingredients for home-cooked meals than they once spent eating out.

Of course there are others way to celebrate than with food, lest you create another food association, and you may want to do that by meeting needs that once triggered emotional eating. You might focus on more fun things to do, more ways to pamper yourself or more time to be with those you love. The more you focus on feeling good, the more you will want to feel your personal best in all facets of your life.

Coaching Questions to

KEEP YOURSELF ON TRACK

How can you remember to be conscious of your hunger levels and check in when you are eating for reasons other than physical hunger?

What is the best way to journal during the week?

What went well this week?

What didn't go so well?

What did you observe about your thoughts or feelings that may help you understand what was driving your behavior?

What do you learn from that?

What did you really need?

What strategy will be most helpful to you if this happens again in the future?

Next Steps

Download Journal Pages

Download the journal pages used by my clients. You may access these freely and as often as you wish. They are available in two formats. One is in a Microsoft Excel format so you can make modifications and tailor it to your own needs. The other is a pdf format that you cannot change but is easier to download and copy for those that don't have or don't feel comfortable with Excel.

> **Fitness journal pages:** www.inspiredtofeelgood.com/journals
>
> **Discovery journal pages:** www.inspiredtofeelgood.com/journals

Get the 9 Life-Changing Secrets and a Connection to Me

Find out more about my story and the nine secrets that changed my life and led me on the journey to writing this book. This is my gift to you. Along with it you will receive a connection to me through my Healthy Living e-newsletter.

Download this special e-book at www.feelyourpersonalbest.com/free_report.asp or visit www.feelyourpersonalbest.com and look for the 9 Secrets banner on the home page.

Listen to *How to Succeed at Living Your Personal Best* Audio Programs

It is one thing to read a book and another to hear concepts presented and questions answered. The *How to Succeed* tele-program series, hosted by me throughout the year, further answers what it takes to address the challenges in making healthy lifestyle changes.

Download the audio recordings of the programs for $16.95 to get more insight about how to achieve your own personal best success. Sign up for the 9 Secrets and Healthy Living e-newsletter to find out about future *How to Succeed* tele-programs.

- How to Conquer Exercise Resistance
- How to Overcome Emotional Eating

- How to End the Diet Mentality

- How to Increase Metabolism

- How to Stay in Control during the Holidays

Go to www.feelyourpersonalbest.com/audio-succeed.asp to learn more about downloading these recordings and to see what new programs have been added, or visit www.feelyourpersonalbest.com and go to the Individuals page for Get Help Audio Programs.

Join a Group Coaching Program or Workshop

Participate in a 16-week group coaching program or 8-week workshop to get assistance putting the concepts of this book into practice. Achieve greater consciousness, clarity and choices to finally reach your goals through facilitated guidance and accountability. Get supported and learn from others as you make changes in your own lifestyle to feel good.

For information about group programs, visit www.feelyourpersonalbest.com/group-coaching.asp or visit www.feelyourpersonalbest.com and go to the Groups page for Coach Guided Groups.

Free Audio

How to Stay Motivated

If you struggle to stay motivated and reach your weight loss, fitness and health goals, then this recording on *How to Stay Motivated* from my tele-program series on How to Succeed on Living Your Personal Best will give you the answer to:

- Why most people can't stay motivated,
- How to tell if you are motivated enough,
- What to avoid to stay on track, and
- The best ways to reach your goals.

Download this free audio to learn the seven ways to avoid giving up on your goals and find out the best way to stay motivated so you can stick with your new fitness and healthy lifestyle changes.

In the audio on *How to Stay Motivated*, you will learn

- The two phases of motivation and how they get you started and keep you going
- Picking goals that drive success for the short and long-term
- How to address life's realities and stay on track
- Redefining what it takes to succeed
- What to really measure so you see progress
- Dealing with disruptions and derailments, so it is easy to get restarted
- Making choices that are so motivating you don't want to stop doing them

Download this free audio recording at www.inspiredtofeelgood.com/audiogift

Appendix

Aerobic Activities

Indoors	Outdoors
Aerobic videos & classes	Biking
Aquatics	Canoeing
Basketball	Chi running or Chi walking
Biking	Cross country skiing
Boxing	Gardening
Dancing	Golf
Dance videos	Hiking and backpacking
Elliptical trainer	Jump rope
Hula hooping	Kayaking
Kickboxing	Nia
Martial arts	Nordic walking
Nia	Race walking
Nordic Trak	Rock climbing
Power Yoga	Roller blading
Racquetball or squash	Running
Rock climbing	Soccer or field hockey
Rowing	Skating
Spinning	Snow shoeing
Stairs	Softball
Swimming & aquatics	Volleyball
Tennis	Walking
Treadmill	Windsurfing

Identifying Your Emotions

Abandoned

Afraid

Aggravated

Alienated

Alone

Angry

Annoyed

Anxious

Apathetic

Apprehensive

Belittled

Betrayed

Bitter

Bored

Burdened

Confused

Depressed

Deprived

Desperate

Discouraged

Disgusted

Distressed

Disturbed

Drained

Embarrassed

Empty

Exasperated

Explosive

Fearful

Frightened

Frustrated

Furious

Helpless

Hesitant

Hopeless

Horrified

Humiliated

Hurt

Impatient

Insecure

Irritated

Isolated

Jealous

Livid

Lonely

Mad

Nervous

Offended

Outraged

Overwhelmed

Pessimistic

Powerless

Pressured

Regretful

Rejected

Remorseful

Resentful

Sad

Shamed

Shattered

Shocked

Smothered

Sorry

Threatened

Trapped

Uncertain

Uncomfortable

Unfulfilled

Unhappy

Upset

Used

Worried

Easy & Fast Recipes

5 Minute Preparation Meals - from my kitchen
Here are several simple, balanced recipes that take about 5 minutes to prepare and anywhere from 15-50 minutes to cook.

Pork tenderloin with sautéed zucchini and yams for 4 (50 minutes)

Ingredients: Pre-marinated pork tenderloin (find a brand and flavor you like)
   4-5 zucchini (you can also do a mix of zucchini and summer squash)
   2 yams (or sweet potatoes)
   ½ tsp dried thyme

- Place pork tenderloin in a low baking pan and bake per directions (about 50 minutes).

   If you want easy clean up, use tin-foil under the pork. You can find recycled tin-foil.

- Thickly slice zucchini and put in a large deep Teflon-coated frying pan or sauté pan (you don't need oil unless you want to add some onion for more flavor). Add a small amount of salt, pepper, thyme to taste. Also add a small amount of water (about ¼ cup) and cover. Periodically stir. It is done when the zucchini become soft.

- Pierce clean yams and put in a microwave-safe container. Microwave for up to 5-6 minutes or until you can easily sink a fork through them. Cover with a light dressing or maple sugar to taste.

<u>Salmon with spinach and basmati rice for 4 (20 minutes)</u>
Ingredients: Large piece of salmon fillet (instead of salmon steaks)
              ½ cup basmati rice
              Bag of 10-oz prewashed spinach
              1 lemon

- Place salmon in a baking or jelly-roll pan, sprinkle with salt and pepper. Squeeze juice over salmon from one whole lemon and let sit for a few minutes. Then put under the broiler for 8-10 minutes (a large jelly roll pan works well). It is done when you can easily slide a fork through the thickest section with no resistance.
  - If you want easy clean up, use tin-foil under the salmon. You can find recycled tin-foil.
- Rinse ½ cup basmati rice and cook for about 15 minutes per directions
- Place clean spinach in a steamer basket set in a pot with enough water underneath and steam for about 5-7 minutes until limp OR put in a large frying pan in batches with 1-2 tablespoons of sesame oil over medium heat to wilt the spinach.

<u>Tilapia with asparagus and brown rice for 4 (15 minutes + time for rice)</u>
Ingredients: 3-4 pieces of tilapia fish
              Bunch of asparagus
              ½ cup uncooked brown rice
              1Tbs of balsamic vinaigrette (I happen to like Lilly's)
              Olive or canola oil

- Sprinkle both sides of tilapia with salt and pepper and pan fry in 1-2 tablespoons of olive or canola oil. Cook first side about 2-3 minutes until the fish turns white about an inch in from the edges. Flip over and cook another 2-3 minutes until you can easily slide a fork through the thickest sections without resistance. Place on serving plates and pour a small amount of balsamic vinaigrette over each piece.
- Clean and trim the ends of the asparagus and place in a deep sauté or frying pan. Add ¼ cup of water and cover. Steam for a few minutes until the water has evaporated and the asparagus is just barely limp. It is better to undercook the asparagus because it will keep cooking after you remove it from the heat. Remove and place asparagus into a dish, and pour 1-2 tablespoons of balsamic vinaigrette on top. Let stand a couple of minutes to absorb the vinaigrette and cool down.
- Serve with brown rice (make as directed in microwave or on the stove). As an option, pour a small amount of balsamic vinaigrette over the rice.

Chicken with pasta and broccoli for 4 (20 minutes)

Ingredients: 4 skinned chicken breasts
2 large broccoli crowns
Whole grain pasta
12-oz can of Italian stewed tomatoes

- Pour can of stewed tomatoes in deep sauté or frying pan and add the chicken breasts. Cover and cook for 5 minutes. Turn the chicken breasts over for another 5 minutes until they feel firm and done.
- Cook pasta per directions.
- Clean broccoli and cut off ends of crowns. Slice length-wise into 5-6 sections or cut off just the florets. Place in a steamer basket set in a pot with enough water underneath and steam for about 10-15 minutes until done.
- Serve chicken with tomato sauce over pasta along with broccoli.

Ham and roasted vegetables for 4 (35 minutes)

Ingredients: Thick slice of lean ham (purchase pre-cooked)
Mix of fresh vegetables (such as broccoli, cauliflower, carrots) cut into chunks
Olive or canola oil
Dried thyme
Salt & pepper

- Put ham on a baking sheet or jelly-roll pan and broil for about 3 minutes per side.
- Place the cut-up raw vegetables on one or more large baking sheets that are already oiled. The fastest way to do this is to spray the pan with oil. I use an oil mister, which is a homemade version of PAM oil sprays.

   If you want easy clean up, use tin-foil under the ham and the vegetables.
- Then spray the vegetables with oil. You can also put the vegetables in a plastic bag with a tablespoon of oil and shake together, before putting the vegetables in the pan.
- Lightly sprinkle dried thyme (or any other spice you like), salt and pepper over the vegetables
- Roast the vegetables at 400 degrees for 20-30 minutes, or until the vegetables start to burn along their edges.

Client Recipes - from Kristen

Warm Greek Spinach Salad for 2 (10 minutes)

Ingredients: 1/2 Bermuda Onion or Vidalia Onion
              1 T. Olive Oil
              10-oz package of baby spinach
              12 cherry or grape tomatoes
              2 oz. low fat feta or goat cheese
              6 Kalamata olives
              Juice of 1/2 lemon
              Freshly ground black pepper

- Sauté the onion in the olive oil until soft and caramelized. Add the spinach to the onions and toss in the hot pan just until warm and a few leaves have wilted. Toss in the feta and tomatoes and olives.
- Serve on large plates. Squeeze 1/4 lemon on each salad and grind fresh pepper on top. This makes a great meal on its own, or top them with some smoked salmon, grilled fish, anchovies, or grilled chicken.

Turkey Chili (20 minutes)

Ingredients: 1 lb ground low fat turkey breast
             2 tbsp olive oil divided
             3 tsp cumin divided
             2 tbsp chili powder divided
             2 cloves garlic, minced
             1 cup diced onion
             1 cup diced bell peppers
             1 cup baby carrots sliced
             32-oz. can diced tomatoes

             salt, pepper, and cayenne to taste

Brown the turkey in a nonstick pan and 1T. olive oil, add 1 tsp. cumin and 1 T. chili powder, salt and pepper.

- Simultaneously sweat the onions, pepper, carrots, and garlic in a large stock pot with the same seasonings.
- When turkey is browned, carefully transfer it into the stockpot and add the tomatoes. Allow to cook until carrots are soft.
- Add cayenne and adjust seasonings to taste.
- For variations, add fresh cilantro and parsley, chopped scallions, or low fat cheese or low fat sour cream. • Serve over brown rice. For efficiency, make a double batch and freeze half-- it'll go fast!

<u>Mediterranean Fish Stew for 4 (30 minutes)</u>
Ingredients: 1 tbsp butter

> 1 tbsp whole wheat flour
> 4 cups cold water
> 6-oz. can of tomato paste
> 15-oz. can of diced tomatoes
> 1 tbsp soy sauce
> 1 tsp dried basil
> 2 tsp dried oregano
> 1 tsp dried thyme
> 1 tsp cumin powder
> 1 tsp cinnamon
> salt and pepper to taste
> 1/2 lb shrimp
> 1/2 lb haddock cubed or white fish cubed or scallops
> 1 cup cooked whole wheat couscous

- Melt the butter in a large soup pot, and add the wheat flour to make a roux. This only takes a few minutes and makes the soup rich and velvety for less than 1 tsp. butter per serving.
- After the roux is medium brown, add the water.
- Whisk in the tomato paste as the water heats, and then add the diced tomatoes and the seasoning.
- Let the soup cook about 15 minutes or as long as you like. (The longer you cook it, the more blended the flavors, but 15 minutes does nicely.)
- During the last 5 minutes, add the fish. This is important to prevent overcooking.
- Put 1/4 c. couscous in each of 4 soup bowls. Ladle the soup over the couscous in 4 equal servings.
- You can add a pinch of cayenne, or hot sauce if you like. Other variations include adding roasted red your own soup, too.

Recommended Resources

Books

Achieving Physical Wealth	by Heather Moreno
Am I Hungry?	by Michelle May, MD
Climb Your Ladder of Success	by John Rowley
Do I Look Fat in This?	by Rhonda Britten
Feel Good Guide to Prosperity	by Eva Gregory
Fries, Thighs & Lies	by Deborah Arneson,
Healing Back Pain	by John Sarno, MD
Intuitive Eating	by Evelyn Tribole, RD & Elyse Resch, RD
Life is Hard, Food is Easy	by Linda Spangle, RD
Living the Truth	by Keith Ablow, MD
My Big Fat Greek Diet	by Nick Yphantides, MD
Soul-full Eating	by Maureen Whitehouse
Teenage Waistland	by Abby Ellin
The Four Day Win	by Martha Beck
The Schwarzbein Principle	by Diana Schwarzbein, MD
Un-Dieting	by Diana Lipson-Burge, RD
Wake Up Inspired	by Marian Baker
You Time	by Asia Sharif-Clark

Publications

Experience Life magazine	www.experiencelifemag.com
Natural Health magazine	www.naturalhealthmag.com
Yoga Journal	www.yogajournal.com

Fitness Products

Collage Video	www.collagevideo.com
Power Systems	www.power-systems.com
Caltrac activity monitor	www.wal-mart.com or www.muscledynamics.com
New-Lifestyles pedometer	www.new-lifestyles.com
Body Bugg activity monitor	www.bodybugg.com
Polar heart rate monitors	www.polarusa.com
Wii interactive exercising	www.nintendo.com/wii

About the Author

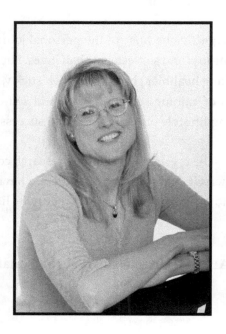

Alice Greene
America's Healthy Lifestyle Coach

Alice knows what it is like to be unhealthy, unfit and overweight. In 2000 she was a size 16, out of shape, and sick with chronic fatigue and digestive issues. During the next two years she discovered how to create and maintain a healthy lifestyle and a positive attitude about taking care of herself that formed the basis of her programs. She continues to be in the best shape of her life and to wear her size 4s, 6s and 8s, knowing it isn't about maintaining a specific size or weight but about being healthy, fit and confident.

Alice has helped hundreds of people discover that food and fitness can truly be an enjoyable and satisfying experience once they let go of their limiting mindset and give themselves permission to make choices that feel good inside and out. She specializes in guiding people to overcome emotional and over eating, conquer exercise resistance, stay motivated and choose healthier options that feel good.

Alice is co-author of *Wake Up Women: Be Happy, Healthy and Wealthy* and the former co-host of the *Living Your Personal Best* talk radio show, which featured healthy lifestyle success stories. She also co-developed the Living Free Diabetes CD program for those with insulin resistance. In addition she speaks, teaches classes and workshops, and conducts private and group coaching.

Clients value Alice's perspective because of the personal journey she took to address her health, fitness, weight-loss and self-esteem challenges. She knows how hard it is to take the first step to making healthier choices and then stick with the changes, and she also knows the freedom of gaining self-confidence and self-esteem that comes from creating a fit and fulfilling lifestyle one small step and success at a time.

In her former life, she was the president of a market research consulting firm and never stopped to take care of herself. Today she is committed to having balance, walking her talk, and being present to experience the precious moments life has to offer.

Contact Alice at agreene@feelyourpersonalbest.com

BUY A SHARE OF THE FUTURE IN YOUR COMMUNITY

These certificates make great holiday, graduation and birthday gifts that can be personalized with the recipient's name. The cost of one S.H.A.R.E. or one square foot is $54.17. The personalized certificate is suitable for framing and will state the number of shares purchased and the amount of each share, as well as the recipient's name. The home that you participate in "building" will last for many years and will continue to grow in value.

Here is a sample SHARE certificate:

THIS CERTIFIES THAT

YOUR NAME HERE

HAS INVESTED IN A HOME FOR A DESERVING FAMILY

1985-2005

TWENTY YEARS OF BUILDING FUTURES IN OUR COMMUNITY ONE HOME AT A TIME

1200 SQUARE FOOT HOUSE @ $65,000 = $54.17 PER SQUARE FOOT
This certificate represents a tax deductible donation. It has no cash value.

YES, I WOULD LIKE TO HELP!

I support the work that Habitat for Humanity does and I want to be part of the excitement! As a donor, I will receive periodic updates on your construction activities but, more importantly, I know my gift will help a family in our community realize the dream of homeownership. **I would like to SHARE in your efforts against substandard housing in my community!** *(Please print below)*

PLEASE SEND ME _____ SHARES at $54.17 EACH = $ $_____

In Honor Of: _____

Occasion: (Circle One)   HOLIDAY   BIRTHDAY   ANNIVERSARY

OTHER: _____

Address of Recipient: _____

Gift From: _____   *Donor Address:* _____

Donor Email: _____

I AM ENCLOSING A CHECK FOR $ $_____ PAYABLE TO HABITAT FOR HUMANITY OR PLEASE CHARGE MY VISA OR MASTERCARD *(CIRCLE ONE)*

Card Number _____   Expiration Date: _____

Name as it appears on Credit Card _____   Charge Amount $ _____

Signature _____

Billing Address _____

Telephone # Day _____   Eve _____

PLEASE NOTE: Your contribution is tax-deductible to the fullest extent allowed by law.
Habitat for Humanity • P.O. Box 1443 • Newport News, VA 23601 • 757-596-5553
www.HelpHabitatforHumanity.org

Printed in the USA
CPSIA information can be obtained
at www.ICGtesting.com
JSHW052016140824
68134JS00027B/2496